An Essay Towards a New Theory

George Berkeley

Table of Contents

An Essay Towards a New Theory..1

George Berkeley...1

AN ESSAY TOWARDS A NEW THEORY OF VISION.....................................1

An Essay Towards a New Theory

George Berkeley

Kessinger Publishing reprints thousands of hard–to–find books!

Visit us at http://www.kessinger.net

AN ESSAY TOWARDS A NEW THEORY OF VISION

1. My design is to show the manner wherein we perceive by sight the distance, magnitude, and situation of OBJECTS. Also to consider the difference there is betwixt the IDEAS of sight and touch, and whether there be any IDEA common to both senses.

2. It is, I think, agreed by all that DISTANCE, of itself and immediately, cannot be seen. For DISTANCE being a Line directed end–wise to the eye, it projects only one point in the fund of the eye, which point remains invariably the same, whether the distance be longer or shorter.

3. I find it also acknowledged that the estimate we make of the distance of OBJECTS considerably remote is rather an act of judgment grounded on EXPERIENCE than of SENSE. For example, when I perceive a great number of intermediate OBJECTS, such as houses, fields, rivers, and the like, which I have experienced to take up a considerable space, I thence form a judgment or conclusion that the OBJECT I see beyond them is at a great distance. Again, when an OBJECT appears faint and small, which at a near distance I have experienced to make a vigorous and large appearance, I instantly conclude it to be far off: And this, it is evident, is the result of EXPERIENCE; without which, from the faintness and littleness I should not have inferred anything concerning the distance of OBJECTS.

4. But when an OBJECT is placed at so near a distance as that the interval between the eyes bears any sensible proportion to it, the opinion of speculative men is that the two

OPTIC AXES (the fancy that we see only with one eye at once being exploded) concurring at the OBJECT do there make an ANGLE, by means of which, according as it is greater or lesser, the OBJECT is perceived to be nearer or farther off.

5. Betwixt which and the foregoing manner of estimating distance there is this remarkable difference: that whereas there was no apparent, necessary connection between small distance and a large and strong appearance, or between great distance and a little and faint appearance, there appears a very necessary connection between an obtuse angle and near distance, and an acute angle and farther distance. It does not in the least depend upon experience, but may be evidently known by anyone before he had experienced it, that the nearer the concurrence of the OPTIC AXES, the greater the ANGLE, and the remoter their concurrence is, the lesser will be the ANGLE comprehended by them.

6. There is another way mentioned by optic writers, whereby they will have us judge of those distances, in respect of which the breadth of the PUPIL hath any sensible bigness: And that is the greater or lesser divergency of the rays, which issuing from the visible point do fall on the PUPIL, that point being judged nearest which is seen by most diverging rays, and that remoter which is seen by less diverging rays: and so on, the apparent distance still increasing, as the divergency of the rays decreases, till at length it becomes infinite, when the rays that fall on the PUPIL are to sense parallel. And after this manner it is said we perceive distance when we look only with one eye.

7. In this case also it is plain we are not beholding to experience: it being a certain, necessary truth that the nearer the direct rays falling on the eye approach to a PARALLELISM, the farther off is the point of their intersection, or the visible point from whence they flow.

8. I have here set down the common, current accounts that are given of our perceiving near distances by sight, which, though they are unquestionably received for true by MATHEMATICIANS, and accordingly made use of by them in determining the apparent places of OBJECTS, do, nevertheless seem to me very unsatisfactory: and that for these following reasons:—

9. FIRST, It is evident that when the mind perceives any IDEA, not immediately and of itself, it must be by the means of some other IDEA. Thus, for instance, the passions which are in the mind of another are of themselves to me invisible. I may nevertheless

perceive them by sight, though not immediately, yet by means of the colours they produce in the countenance. We often see shame or fear in the looks of a man, by perceiving the changes of his countenance to red or pale.

10. Moreover it is evident that no IDEA which is not itself perceived can be the means of perceiving any other IDEA. If I do not perceive the redness or paleness of a man's face themselves, it is impossible I should perceive by them the passions which are in his mind.

11. Now from sect. 2 it is plain that distance is in its own nature imperceptible, and yet it is perceived by sight. It remains, therefore, that it be brought into view by means of some other IDEA that is itself immediately perceived in the act of VISION.

12. But those LINES and ANGLES, by means whereof some MATHEMATICIANS pretend to explain the perception of distance, are themselves not at all perceived, nor are they in truth ever thought of by those unskilful in optics. I appeal to anyone's experience whether upon sight of an OBJECT he computes its distance by the bigness of the ANGLE made by the meeting of the two OPTIC AXES? Or whether he ever thinks of the greater or lesser divergency of the rays, which arrive from any point to his PUPIL? Everyone is himself the best judge of what he perceives, and what not. in vain shall all the MATHEMATICIANS in the world tell me, that I perceive certain LINES and ANGLES which introduce into my mind the various IDEAS of DISTANCE, so long as I myself am conscious of no such thing.

13. Since, therefore, those ANGLES and LINES are not themselves perceived by sight, it follows from sect. 10 that the mind doth not by them judge of the distance of OBJECTS.

14. Secondly, the truth of this assertion will be yet farther evident to anyone that considers those LINES and ANGLES have no real existence in nature, being only an HYPOTHESIS framed by the MATHEMATICIANS, and by them introduced into OPTICS, that they might treat of that science in a GEOMETRICAL way.

15. The third and last reason I shall give for rejecting that doctrine is, that though we should grant the real existence of those OPTIC ANGLES, etc., and that it was possible for the mind to perceive them, yet these principles would not be found sufficient to explain the PHENOMENA of DISTANCE, as shall be shown hereafter.

16. Now, it being already shown that distance is suggested to the mind by the mediation of some other IDEA which is itself perceived in the act of seeing, it remains that we inquire what IDEAS or SENSATIONS there be that attend VISION, unto which we may suppose the IDEAS of distance are connected, and by which they are introduced into the mind. And FIRST, it is certain by experience that when we look at a near OBJECT with both eyes, according as it approaches or recedes from us, we alter the disposition of our eyes, by lessening or widening the interval between the PUPILS. This disposition or turn of the eyes is attended with a sensation, which seems to me to be that which in this case brings the IDEA of greater or lesser distance into the mind.

17. Not that there is any natural or necessary connection between the sensation we perceive by the turn of the eyes and greater or lesser distance, but because the mind has by constant EXPERIENCE found the different sensations corresponding to the different dispositions of the eyes to be attended each with a different degree of distance in the OBJECT: there has grown an habitual or customary connection between those two sorts of IDEAS, so that the mind no sooner perceives the sensation arising from the different turn it gives the eyes, In order to bring the PUPILS nearer or farther asunder, but it withal perceives the different IDEA of distance which was wont to be connected with that sensation; just as upon hearing a certain sound, the IDEA is immediately suggested to the understanding which custom had united with it.

18 Nor do I see how I can easily be mistaken in this matter. I know evidently that distance is not perceived of itself. That by consequence it must be perceived by means of some other IDEA which is immediately perceived, and varies with the different degrees of distance. I know also that the sensation arising from the turn of the eyes is of itself immediately perceived, and various degrees thereof are connected with different distances, which never fail to accompany them into my mind, when I view an OBJECT distinctly with both eyes, whose distance is so small that in respect of it the interval between the eyes has any considerable magnitude.

19. I know it is a received opinion that by altering the disposition of the eyes the mind perceives whether the angle of the OPTIC AXES is made greater or lesser. And that accordingly by a kind of NATURAL GEOMETRY it judges the point of their intersection to be nearer or farther off. But that this is not true I am convinced by my own experience, since I am not conscious that I make any such use of the perception I have by the turn of my eyes. And for me to make those judgments, and draw those conclusions

from it, without knowing that I do so, seems altogether incomprehensible.

20. From all which it follows that the judgment we make of the distance of an OBJECT, viewed with both eyes, is entirely the RESULT OF EXPERIENCE. If we had not constantly found certain sensations arising from the various disposition of the eyes, attended with certain degrees of distance, we should never make those sudden judgments from them concerning the distance of OBJECTS; no more than we would pretend to judge a man's thoughts by his pronouncing words we had never heard before.

21. Secondly, an OBJECT placed at a certain distance from the eye, to which the breadth of the PUPIL bears a considerable proportion, being made to approach, is seen more confusedly: and the nearer it is brought the more confused appearance it makes. And this being found constantly to be so, there ariseth in the mind an habitual CONNECTION between the several degrees of confusion and distance; the greater confusion still implying the lesser distance, and the lesser confusion the greater distance of the OBJECT.

22. This confused appearance of the OBJECT doth therefore seem to be the MEDIUM whereby the mind judgeth of distance in those cases wherein the most approved writers of optics will have it judge by the different divergency with which the rays flowing from the radiating point fall on the PUPIL. No man, I believe, will pretend to see or feel those imaginary angles that the rays are supposed to form according to their various inclinations on his eye. But he cannot choose seeing whether the OBJECT appear more or less confused. It is therefore a manifest consequence from what bath been demonstrated, that instead of the greater or lesser divergency of the rays, the mind makes use of the greater or lesser confusedness of the appearance, thereby to determine the apparent place of an OBJECT.

23 Nor doth it avail to say there is not any necessary connection between confused VISION and distance, great or small. For I ask any man what necessary connection he sees between the redness of a blush and shame? And yet no sooner shall he behold that colour to arise in the face of another, but it brings into his and the IDEA of that passion which hath been observed to accompany it.

24. What seems to have misled the writers of optics in this matter is that they imagine men judge of distance as they do of a conclusion in mathematics, betwixt which and the

premises it is indeed absolutely requisite there be an apparent, necessary connection: but it is far otherwise in the sudden judgments men make of distance. We are not to think that brutes and children, or even grown reasonable men, whenever they perceive an OBJECT to approach, or depart from them, do it by virtue of GEOMETRY and DEMONSTRATION.

25. That one IDEA may suggest another to the mind it will suffice that they have been observed to go together, without any demonstration of the necessity of their coexistence, or without so much as knowing what it is that makes them so to coexist. Of this there are innumerable instances of which no one can be ignorant.

26. Thus, greater confusion having been constantly attended with nearer distance, no sooner is the former IDEA perceived, but it suggests the latter to our thoughts. And if it had been the ordinary course of Nature that the farther off an OBJECT were placed, the more confused it should appear, it is certain the very same perception that now makes us think an OBJECT approaches would then have made us to imagine it went farther off. That perception, abstracting from CUSTOM and EXPERIENCE, being equally fitted to produce the IDEA of great distance, or small distance, or no distance at all.

27. Thirdly, an OBJECT being placed at the distance above specified, and brought nearer to the eye, we may nevertheless prevent, at least for some time, the appearances growing more confused, by straining the eye. In which case that sensation supplies the place of confused VISION in aiding the mind to judge of the distance of the OBJECT; it being esteemed so much the nearer by how much the effort or straining of the eye in order to distinct VISION is greater.

28. I have here set down those sensations or IDEAS that seem to be the constant and general occasions of introducing into the mind the different IDEAS of near distance. It is true in most cases that divers other circumstances contribute to frame our IDEA of distance, to wit, the particular number, size, kind, etc., of the things seen. Concerning which, as well as all other the forementioned occasions which suggest distance, I shall only observe they have none of them, in their own nature, any relation or connection with it: nor is it possible they should ever signify the various degrees thereof, otherwise than as by EXPERIENCE they have been found to be connected with them.

29. I shall proceed upon these principles to account for a phenomenon which has hitherto strangely puzzled the writers of optics, and is so far from being accounted for by any of their THEORIES OF VISION that it is, by their own confession, plainly repugnant to them; and of consequence, if nothing else could be objected, were alone sufficient to bring their credit in question. The whole difficulty I shall lay before you in the words of the learned Dr. Barrow, with which he concludes his optic lectures:—

'I have here delivered what my thoughts have suggested to me concerning that part of optics which is more properly mathematical. As for the other parts of that science (which being rather physical, do consequently abound with plausible conjectures instead of certain principles), there has in them scarce anything occurred to my observation different from what has been already said by Kepler, Scheinerus, Descartes, and others. And methinks, I had better say nothing at all, than repeat that which has been so often said by others. I think it therefore high time to take my leave of this subject: but before I quit it for good and all, the fair and ingenuous dealing that I owe both to you and to truth obligeth me to acquaint you with a certain untoward difficulty, which seems directly opposite to the doctrine I have been hitherto inculcating, at least, admits of no solution from it. In short it is this. Before the double convex glass or concave speculum EBF, let the point A be placed at such a distance that the rays proceeding from A, after refraction or reflection, be brought to unite somewhere in the AxAB. And suppose the point of union (i.e. the image of the point A, as hath been already set forth) to be Z; between which and B, the vertex of the glass or speculum, conceive the eye to be anywhere placed. The question now is, where the point A ought to appear? Experience shows that it does not appear behind at the point Z, and it were contrary to nature that it should, since all the impression which affects the sense comes from towards A. But from our tenets it should seem to follow that it would appear before the eye at a vast distance off, so great as should in some sort surpass all sensible distance. For since if we exclude all anticipations and prejudices, every OBJECT appears by so much the farther off, by how much the rays it sends to the eye are less diverging. And that OBJECT is thought to be most remote from which parallel rays proceed unto the eye. Reason would make one think that OBJECT should appear at yet a greater distance which is seen by converging rays. Moreover it may in general be asked concerning this case what it is that determines the apparent place of the point A, and maketh it to appear after a constant manner sometimes nearer, at other times farther off? To which doubt I see nothing that can be answered agreeable to the principles we have laid down except only that the point A ought always to appear extremely remote. But on the contrary we are assured by experience that the point A appears variously distant, according to the different situations of the eye between the points B and Z. And that it doth never (if at all) seem farther off, than it would if it were beheld by the naked eye, but on the contrary it doth sometimes appear much nearer. Nay, it is even certain that by how much the rays falling on the eye do more converge by so much the nearer doth the OBJECT seem to approach. For the eye being placed close to the point B, the OBJECT A appears nearly in its own natural place, if the point B is taken in the glass, or at the same distance, if in the speculum. The eye being brought back to O, the OBJECT seems to draw near: and being come to P it beholds it still nearer. And so on little and little, till at length the eye being placed somewhere, suppose at Q, the OBJECT appearing extremely near, begins to vanish into mere confusion. All which doth seem repugnant to our principles, at least not rightly to agree with them. Nor is our tenet alone struck at by this experiment, but likewise all others that ever came to my knowledge are, every whit as much, endangered by it. The ancient one especially (which is most commonly received, and comes nearest to mine) seems to be so effectually overthrown thereby that the most learned Tacquet has been forced to reject that principle, as false and uncertain, on which alone he had built almost his whole CATOPTRICS; and consequently by taking away the foundation, hath himself pulled down the superstructure he had raised on it. Which, nevertheless, I do not believe he would have done had he but considered the whole matter more thoroughly, and examined the difficulty to the bottom. But as for me, neither this nor any other difficulty shall have so great an influence on me as to make me renounce that which I know to be manifestly agreeable to reason: especially when, as it here falls out, the difficulty is founded in the peculiar nature of a certain odd and particular case. For in the present case something peculiar lies hid, which being involved in the subtilty of nature will, perhaps, hardly be discovered till such time as the manner of vision is more perfectly made known. Concerning which, I must own, I have hitherto been able to find out nothing that has the least show of PROBABILITY, not to mention CERTAINTY. I shall, therefore, leave this knot to be untied by you, wishing you may have better success in it than I have had.'

30. The ancient and received principle, which Dr. Barrow here mentions as the main foundation of Tacquet's CATOPTRICS, is that: 'every visible point seen by reflection from a speculum shall appear placed at the intersection of the reflected ray, and the perpendicular of incidence:' which intersection in the present case, happening to be behind the eye, it greatly shakes the authority of that principle, whereon the aforementioned author proceeds throughout his whole CATOPTRICS in determining the

apparent place of OBJECTS seen by reflection from any kind of speculum.

31. Let us now see how this phenomenon agrees with our tenets. The eye the nearer it is placed to the point B in the foregoing figures, the more distinct is the appearance of the OBJECT; but as it recedes to O the appearance grows more confused; and at P it sees the OBJECT yet more confused; and so on till the eye being brought back to Z sees the OBJECT in the greatest confusion of all. Wherefore by sect. 21 the OBJECT should seem to approach the eye gradually as it recedes from the point B, that is, at O it should (in consequence of the principle I have laid down in the aforesaid section) seem nearer than it did at B, and at P nearer than at 0, and at Q nearer than at P; and so on, till it quite vanishes at Z. Which is the very matter of fact, as anyone that pleases may easily satisfy himself by experiment.

32. This case is much the same as if we should suppose an Englishman to meet a foreigner who used the same words with the English, but in a direct contrary signification. The Englishman would not fail to make a wrong judgment of the IDEAS annexed to those sounds in the mind of him that used them. Just so, in the present case the OBJECT speaks (if I may so say) with words that the eye is well acquainted with, that is, confusions of appearance; but whereas heretofore the greater confusions were always wont to signify nearer distances, they have in this case a direct, contrary signification, being connected with the greater distances. Whence it follows that the eye must unavoidably be mistaken, since it will take the confusions in the sense it has been used to, which is directly opposed to the true.

33. This phenomenon as it entirely subverts the opinion of those who will have us judge of distance by lines and angles, on which supposition it is altogether inexplicable, so it seems to me no small confirmation of the truth of that principle whereby it is explained. But in order co a more full explication of this point, and to show how far the hypothesis of the mind's judging by the various divergency of rays may be of use in determining the apparent place of an OBJECT, it will be necessary to premise some few things, which are already well known to those who have any skill in dioptrics.

34. FIRST, any radiating point is then distinctly seen when the rays proceeding from it are, by the refractive power of the crystalline, accurately reunited in the retina or fund of the eye: but if they are reunited, either before they arrive at the retina, or after they have passed it, then there is confused vision.

35. SECONDLY, suppose in the adjacent figures NP represent an eye duly framed and retaining its natural figure. In Fig. 1 the rays falling nearly parallel on the eye, are by the crystalline AB refracted, so as their focus or point of union F falls exactly on the retina: but if the rays fall sensibly diverging on the eye, as in Fig. 2, then their focus falls beyond the retina: or if the rays are made to converge by the lens QS before they come at the eye, as in Fig. 3, their focus F will fall before the retina. In which two last cases it is evident from the foregoing section that the appearance of the point Z is confused. And by how much the greater is the convergency, or divergency, of the rays falling on the pupil, by so much the farther will the point of their reunion be from the retina, either before or behind it, and consequently the point Z will appear by so much the more confused. And this, by the bye, may show us the difference between confused and faint vision. Confused vision is when the rays proceedings from each distinct point of the OBJECT are not accurately recollected in one corresponding point on the retina, but take up some space thereon, so that rays from different points become mixed and confused together. This is opposed to a distinct vision, and attends near objects. Faint vision is when by reason of the distance of the object or grossness of the interjacent medium few rays arrive from the object to the eye. This is opposed to vigorous or clear vision, and attends remote objects. But to return.

36. The eye, or (to speak truly) the mind, perceiving only the confusion itself, without ever considering the cause from which it proceeds, doth constantly annex the same degree of distance to the same degree of confusion. Whether that confusion be occasioned by converging or by diverging rays, it matters not. Whence it follows that the eye viewing the object Z through the glass QS (which by refraction causeth the rays ZQ, ZS, etc., to converge) should judge it to be at such a nearness at which if it were placed it would radiate on the eye with rays diverging to that degree as would produce the same confusion which is now produced by converging rays, i.e. would cover a portion of the retina equal to DC (VID. Fig. 3 supra). But then this must be understood (to use Dr. Barrow's phrase) SECLUSIS PRAENOTIONIBUS ET PRAEJUDICIIS, in case we abstract from all other circumstances of vision, such as the figure, size, faintness, etc. of the visible objects; all which do ordinarily concur to form our idea of distance, the mind having by frequent experience observed their several sorts or degrees to be conneted with various distances.

37 It plainly follows from what hath been said that a person perfectly purblind (i.e. that could not see an object distinctly but when placed close to his eye) would not make the same wrong judgment that others do in the forementioned case. For to him greater

confusions constantly suggesting greater distances, he must, as he recedes from the glass and the object grows more confused, judge it to be at a farther distance, contrary to what they do who have had the perception of the objects growing more confused connected with the idea of approach.

38. Hence also it doth appear there may be good use of computation by lines and angles in optics; not that the mind judgeth of distance immediately by them, but because it judgeth by somewhat which is connected with them, and to the determination whereof they may be subservient. Thus the mind judging of the distance of an object by the confusedness of its appearance, and this confusedness being greater or lesser to the naked eye, according as the object is seen by rays more or less diverging, it follows that a man may make use of the divergency of the rays in computing the apparent distance, though not for its own sake, yet on account of the confusion with which it is connected. But, so it is, the confusion itself is entirely neglected by mathematicians as having no necessary relation with distance, such as the greater or lesser angles of divergency are conceived to have. And these (especially for that they fall under mathematical computation) are alone regarded in determining the apparent places of objects, as though they were the sole and immediate cause of the judgments the mind makes of distance. Whereas, in truth, they should not at all be regarded in themselves, or any otherwise, than as they are supposed to be the cause of confused vision.

39. The not considering of this has been a fundamental and perplexing oversight. For proof whereof we need go no farther than the case before us. It having been observed that the most diverging rays brought into the mind the idea of nearest distance, and that still, as the divergency decreased, the distance increased: and it being thought the connexion between the various degrees of divergency and distance was immediate; this naturally leads one to conclude, from an ill–grounded analogy, that converging rays shall make an object appear at an immense distance: and that, as the convergency increases, the distance (if it were possible) should do so likewise. That this was the cause of Dr. Barrow's mistake is evident from his own words which we have quoted. Whereas had the learned doctor observed that diverging and converging rays, how opposite soever they may seem, do nevertheless agree in producing the same effect, to wit, confusedness of vision, greater degrees whereof are produced indifferently, either as the divergency or convergency and the rays increaseth. And that it is by this effect, which is the same in both, that either the divergency or convergency is perceived by the eye; I say, had he but considered this, it is certain he would have made a quite contrary judgment, and rightly concluded that those

rays which fall on the eye with greater degrees of convergency should make the object from whence they proceed appear by so much the nearer. But it is plain it was impossible for any man to attain to a right notion of this matter so long as he had regard only to lines and angles, and did not apprehend the true nature of vision, and how far it was of mathematical consideration.

40. Before we dismiss this subject, it is fit we take notice of a query relating thereto, proposed by the ingenious Mr. Molyneux, is his TREATISE OF DIOPTRICS,[Par. I. Prop. 31, Sect. 9.] where speaking of this difficulty, he has these words: 'And so he (i.e. Dr. Barrow) leaves this difficulty to the solution of others, which I (after so great an example) shall do likewise; but with the resolution of the same admirable author of not quitting the evident doarine which we have before laid down, for determining the LOCUS OBJECTI, on account of being pressed by one difficulty which seems inexplicable till a more intimate knowledge of the visive faculty be obtained by mortals. In the meantime, I propose it to the consideration of the ingenious, whether the LOCUS APPARENS of an object placed as in this 9th section be not as much before the eye as the distinct base is behind the eye!' To which query we may venture to answer in the negative. For in the present case the rule for determining the distance of the distinct base, or respective focus from the glass, is this: as the difference between the distance of the object and focus is to the focus or focal length, so the distance of the object from the glass is to the distance of the respective focus or distinct base from the glass. [Molyneux Dioptr., Par. I. Prop. 5.] Let us now suppose the object to be placed at the distance of the focal length, and one half of the focal length from the glass, and the eye close to the glass, hence it will follow by the rule that the distance of the distinct base behind the eye is double the true distance of the object before the eye. If therefore Mr. Molyneux's conjecture held good, it would follow that the eye should see the object twice as far off as it really is; and in other cases at three or four times its due distance, or more. But this manifestly contradicts experience, the object never appearing, at farthest, beyond its due distance. Whatever, therefore, is built on this supposition (VID. COROL. I. PROP. 57, IBID.) comes to the ground along with it.

41. From what hath been premised it is a manifest consequence that a man born blind, being made to see, would, at first, have no idea of distance by sight; the sun and stars, the remotest objects as well as the nearer, would all seem to be in his eye, or rather in his mind. The objects intromitted by sight would seem to him (as in truth they are) no other than a new set of thoughts or sensations, each whereof is as near to him as the perceptions

of pain or pleasure, or the most inward passions of his soul. For our judging objects provided by sight to be at any distance, or without the mind, is (VID. sect. 28) entirely the effect of experience, which one in those circumstances could not yet have attained to.

42. It is indeed otherwise upon the common supposition that men judge of distance by the angle of the optic axes, just as one in the dark, or a blind-man by the angle comprehended by two sticks, one whereof he held in each hand. For if this were true, it would follow that one blind from his birth being made to see, should stand in need of no new experience in order to perceive distance by sight. But that this is false has, I think, been sufficiently demonstrated.

43. And perhaps upon a strict inquiry we shall not find that even those who from their birth have grown up in a continued habit of seeing are irrecoverably prejudiced on the other side, to wit, in thinking what they see to be at a distance from them. For at this time it seems agreed on all hands, by those who have had any thoughts of that matter, that colours, which are the proper and immediate object of sight, are not without the mind. But then it will be said, by sight we have also the ideas of extension, and figure, and motion; all which may well be thought without, and at some distance from the mind, though colour should not. In answer to this I appeal to any man's experience, whether the visible extension of any object doth not appear as near to him as the colour of that object; nay, whether they do not both seem to be in the very same place. Is not the extension we see coloured, and is it possible for us, so much as in thought, to separate and abstract colour from extension? Now, where the extension is there surely is the figure, and there the motion too. I speak of those which are perceived by sight.

44. But for a fuller explication of this point, and to show that the immediate objects of sight are not so much as the ideas or resemblances of things placed at a distance, it is requisite that we look nearer into the matter and carefully observe what is meant in common discourse, when one says that which he sees is at a distance from him. Suppose, for example, that looking at the moon I should say it were fifty or sixty semidiameters of the earth distant from me. Let us see what moon this is spoken of: it is plain it cannot be the visible moon, or anything like the visible moon, or that which I see, which is only a round, luminous plane of about thirty visible points in diameter. For in case I am carried from the place where I stand directly towards the moon, it is manifest the object varies, still as I go on; and by the time that I am advanced fifty or sixty semidiameters of the earth, I shall be so far from being near a small, round, luminous flat that I shall perceive

13

nothing like it; this object having long since disappeared, and if I would recover it, it must be by going back to the earth from whence I set out. Again, suppose I perceive by sight the faint and obscure idea of something which I doubt whether it be a man, or a tree, or a tower, but judge it to be at the distance of about a mile. It is plain I cannot mean that what I see is a mile off, or that it is the image or likeness of anything which is a mile off, since that every step I take towards it the appearance alters, and from being obscure, small, and faint, grows clear, large, and vigorous. And when I come to the mile's end, that which I saw first is quite lost, neither do I find anything in the likeness of it.

45. In these and the like instances the truth of the matter stands thus: having of a long time experienced certain ideas, perceivable by touch, as distance, tangible figure, and solidity, to have been connected with certain ideas of sight, I do upon perceiving these ideas of sight forthwith conclude what tangible ideas are, by the wonted ordinary course of Nature like to follow. Looking at an object I perceive a certain visible figure and colour, with some degree of faintness and other circumstances, which from what I have formerly observed, determine me to think that if I advance forward so many paces or miles, I shall be affected with such and such ideas of touch: so that in truth and strictness of speech I neither see distance itself, nor anything that I take to be at a distance. I say, neither distance nor things placed at a distance are themselves, or their ideas, truly perceived by sight. This I am persuaded of, as to what concerns myself: and I believe whoever will look narrowly into his own thoughts and examine what he means by saying he sees this or that thing at a distance, will agree with me that what he sees only suggests to his understanding that after having passed a certain distance, to be measured by the motion of his body, which is perceivable by touch, he shall come to perceive such and such tangible ideas which have been usually connected with such and such visible ideas. But that one might be deceived by these suggestions of sense, and that there is no necessary connexion between visible and tangible ideas suggested by them, we need go no farther than the next looking–glass or pictures to be convinced. Note that when I speak of tangible ideas, I take the word idea for any the immediate object of sense or understanding, in which large signification it is commonly used by the moderns.

46. From what we have shown it is a manifest consequence that the ideas of space, outness, and things placed at a distance are not, strictly speaking, the object of sight; they are not otherwise perceived by the eye than by the ear. Sitting in my study I hear a coach drive along the street; I look through the casement and see it; I walk out and enter into it; thus, common speech would incline one to think I heard, saw, and touched the same

thing, to wit, the coach. It is nevertheless certain, the ideas intromitted by each sense are widely different and distinct from each other; but having been observed constantly to go together, they are spoken of as one and the same thing. By the variation of the noise I perceive the different distances of the coach, and know that it approaches before I look out. Thus by the ear I perceive distance, just after the same manner as I do by the eye.

47. I do not nevertheless say I hear distance in like manner as I say that I see it, the ideas perceived by hearing not being so apt to be confounded with the ideas of touch as those of sight are. So likewise a man is easily convinced that bodies and external things are not properly the object of hearing; but only sounds, by the mediation whereof the idea of this or that body or distance is suggested to his thoughts. But then one is with more difficulty brought to discern the difference there is betwixt the ideas of sight and touch: though it be certain a man no more sees and feels the same thing than he hears and feels the same thing.

48. One reason of which seems to be this. It is thought a great absurdity to imagine that one and the same thing should have any more than one extension, and one figure. But the extension and figure of a body, being let into the mind two ways, and that indifferently either by sight or touch, it seems to follow that we see the same extension and the same figure which we feel.

49. But if we take a close and accurate view of things, it must be acknowledged that we never see and feel one and the same object. That which is seen is one thing, and that which is felt is another. If the visible figure and extension be not the same with the tangible figure and extension, we are not to infer that one and the same thing has divers extensions. The true consequence is that the objects of sight and touch are two distinct things. It may perhaps require some thought rightly to conceive this distinction. And the difficulty seems not a little increased, because the combination of visible ideas hath constantly the same name as the combination of tangible ideas wherewith it is connected: which doth of necessity arise from the use and end of language.

50. In order therefore to treat accurately and unconfusedly of vision, we must bear in mind that there are two sorts of objects apprehended by the eye, the one primarily and immediately, the other secondarily and by intervention of the former. Those of the first sort neither are, nor appear to be, without the mind, or at any distance off; they may indeed grow greater or smaller, more confused, or more clear, or more faint, but they do

not, cannot approach or recede from us. Whenever we say an object is at a distance, whenever we say it draws near, or goes farther off, we must always mean it of the latter sort, which properly belong to the touch, and are not so truly perceived as suggested by the eye in like manner as thoughts by the ear.

51. No sooner do we hear the words of a familiar language pronounced in our ears, but the ideas corresponding thereto present themselves to our minds: in the very same instant the sound and the meaning enter the understanding: so closely are they united that it is not in our power to keep out the one, except we exclude the other also. We even act in all respects as if we heard the very thoughts themselves. So likewise the secondary objects, or those which are only suggested by sight, do often more strongly affect us, and are more regarded than the proper objects of that sense; along with which they enter into the mind, and with which they have a far more strict connexion, than ideas have with words. Hence it is we find it so difficult to discriminate between the immediate and mediate objects of sight, and are so prone to attribute to the former what belongs only to the latter. They are, as it were, most closely twisted, blended, and incorporated together. And the prejudice is confirmed and riveted in our thoughts by a long tract of time, by the use of language, and want of reflexion. However, I believe anyone that shall attentively consider what we have already said, and shall say, upon this subject before we have done (especially if he pursue it in his own thoughts) may be able to deliver himself from that prejudice. Sure I am it is worth some attention, to whoever would understand the true nature of vision.

52. I have now done with distance, and proceed to show how it is that we perceive by sight the magnitude of objects. It is the opinion of some that we do it by angles, or by angles in conjunction with distance: but neither angles nor distance being perceivable by sight, and the things we see being in truth at no distance from us, it follows that as we have shown lines and angles not to be the medium the mind makes use of in apprehending the apparent place, so neither are they the medium whereby it apprehends the apparent magnitude of objects.

53. It is well known that the same extension at a near distance shall subtend a greater angle, and at a farther distance a lesser angle. And by this principle (we are told) the mind estimates the magnitude of an object, comparing the angle under which it is seen with its distance, and thence inferring the magnitude thereof. What inclines men to this mistake (beside the humour of making one see by geometry)is that the same perceptions or ideas

16

which suggest distance do also suggest magnitude. But if we examine it we shall find they suggest the latter as immediately as the former. I say, they do not first suggest distance, and then leave it to the judgment to use that as a medium whereby to collect the magnitude; but they have as close and immediate a connexion with the magnitude as with the distance; and suggest magnitude as independently of distance as they do distance independently of magnitude. All which will be evident to whoever considers what hath been already said, and what follows.

54. It hath been shown there are two sorts of objects apprehended by sight; each whereof hath its distinct magnitude, or extension. The one, properly tangible, i.e. to be perceived and measured by touch, and not immediately falling under the sense of seeing: the other, properly and immediately visible, by mediation of which the former is brought in view. Each of these magnitudes are greater or lesser, according as they contain in them more or fewer points, they being made up of points or minimums. For, whatever may be said of extension in abtract, it is certain sensible extension is not infinitely divisible. There is a MINIMUM TANGIBILE and a MINIMUM VISIBILE, beyond which sense cannot perceive. This everyone's experience will inform him.

55. The magnitude of the object which exists without the mind, and is at a distance, continues always invariably the same: but the visible object still changing as you approach to, or recede from, the tangible object, it hath no fixed and determinate greatness. Whenever, therefore, we speak of the magnitude of anything, for instance a tree or a house, we must mean the tangible magnitude, otherwise there can be nothing steady and free from ambiguity spoken of it. But though the tangible and visible magnitude in truth belong to two distinct objects: I shall nevertheless (especially since those objects are called by the same name, and are observed to coexist), to avoid tediousness and singularity of speech, sometimes speak of them as belonging to one and the same thing.

56. Now in order to discover by what means the magnitude of tangible objects is perceived by sight. I need only reflect on what passes in my own mind, and observe what those things be which introduce the ideas of greater or lesser into my thoughts, when I look on any object. And these I find to be, FIRST, the magnitude or extension of the visible object, which being immediately perceived by sight, is connected with that other which is tangible and placed at a distance. SECONDLY, the confusion or distinctness. And thirdly, the vigorousness or faintness of the aforesaid visible appearance. CETERIS

PARIBUS, by how much the greater or lesser the visible object is, by so much the greater or lesser do I conclude the tangible object to be. But, be the idea immediately perceived by sight never so large, yet if it be withal confused, I judge the magnitude of the thing to be but small. If it be distinct and clear, I judge it greater. And if it be faint, I apprehend it to be yet greater. What is here meant by confusion and faintness hath been explained in sect. 35.

57. Moreover the judgments we make of greatness do, in like manner as those of distance, depend on the disposition of the eye, also on the figure, number, and situation of objects and other circumstances that have been observed to attend great or small tangible magnitudes. Thus, for instance, the very same quantity of visible extension, which in the figure of a tower doth suggest the idea of great magnitude, shall in the figure of a man suggest the idea of much smaller magnitude. That this is owing to the experience we have had of the usual bigness of a tower and a man no one, I suppose, need be told.

58. It is also evident that confusion or faintness have no more a necessary connexion with little or great magnitude than they have with little or great distance. As they suggest the latter, so they suggest the former to our minds. And by consequence, if it were not for experience, we should no more judge a faint or confused appearance to be connected with great or little magnitude, than we should that it was connected with great or little distance.

59. Nor will it be found that great or small visible magnitude hath any necessary relation to great or small tangible magnitude: so that the one may certainly be inferred from the other. But before we come to the proof of this, it is fit we consider the difference there is betwixt the extension and figure which is the proper object of touch, and that other which is termed visible; and how the former is principally, though not immediately taken notice of, when we look at any object. This has been before mentioned, but we shall here inquire into the cause thereof. We regard the objects that environ us in proportion as they are adapted to benefit or injure our own bodies, and thereby produce in our minds the sensation of pleasure or pain. Now bodies operating on our organs, by an immediate application, and the hurt or advantage arising therefrom, depending altogether on the tangible, and not at all on the visible, qualities of any object: this is a plain reason why those should be regarded by us much more than these: and for this end the visive sense seems to have been bestowed on animals, to wit, that by the perception of visible ideas (which in themselves are not capable of affecting or any wise altering the frame of their

bodies) they may be able to foresee (from the experience they have had what tangible ideas are connected with such and such visible ideas) and damage or benefit which is like to ensue, upon the application of their own bodies to this or that body which is at a distance. Which foresight, how necessary it is to the preservation of an animal, everyone's experience can inform him. Hence it is that when we look at an object, the tangible figure and extension thereof are principally attended to; whilst there is small heed taken of the visible figure and magnitude, which, though more immediately perceived, do less concern us, and are not fitted to produce any alteration in our bodies.

60. That the matter of fact is true will be evident to anyone who considers that a man placed at ten foot distance is thought as great as if he were placed at a distance only of five foot: which is true not with relation to the visible, but tangible greatness of the object: the visible magnitude being far greater at one station: than it is at the other.

61. Inches, feet, etc., are settled stated lengths whereby we measure objects and estimate their magnitude: we say, for example, an object appears to be six inches or six foot long. Now, that this cannot be meant of visible inches, etc., is evident, because a visible inch is itself no constant, determinate magnitude, and cannot therefore serve to mark out and determine the magnitude of any other thing. Take an inch marked upon a ruler: view it, successively, at the distance of half a foot, a foot, a foot and a half, etc., from the eye: at each of which, and at all the intermediate distances, the inch shall have a different visible extension, i.e. there shall be more or fewer points discerned in it. Now I ask which of all these various extensions is that stated, determinate one that is agreed on for a common measure of other magnitudes? No reason can be assigned why we should pitch on one more than another: and except there be some invariable, determinate extension fixed on to be marked to the word inch, it is plain it can be used to little purpose; and to say a thing contains this or that number of inches shall imply no more than that it is extended, without bringing any particular idea of that extension into the mind. Farther, an inch and a foot, from different distances, shall both exhibit the same visible magnitude, and yet at the same time you shall say that one seems several times greater than the other. From all which it is manifest that the judgments we make of the magnitude of objects by sight are altogether in reference to their tangible extension. Whenever we say an object is great, or small, of this or that determinate measure, I say it must be meant of the tangible, and not the visible extension, which, though immediately perceived, is nevertheless little taken notice of.

62. Now, that there is no necessary connexion between these two distinct extensions is evident from hence: because our eyes might have been framed in such a manner as to be able to see nothing but what were less than the MINIMUM TANGIBILE. In which case it is not impossible we might have perceived all the immediate objects of sight, the very same that we do now: but unto those visible appearances there would not be connected those different tangible magnitudes that are now. Which shows the judgments we make of the magnitude of things placed at a distance from the various greatness of the immediate objects of sight do not arise from any essential or necessary but only a customary tie, which has been observed between them.

63. Moreover, it is not only certain that any idea of sight might not have been connected with this or that idea of touch, which we now observe to accompany it: but also that the greater visible magnitudes might have been connected with, and introduced into our minds lesser tangible magnitudes and the lesser visible magnitudes greater tangible magnitudes. Nay, that it actually is so we have daily experience; that object which makes a strong and large appearance, not seeming near so great as another, the visible magnitude whereof is much less, but more faint, and the appearance upper, or which is the same thing painted lower on the RETINA, which faintness and situation suggest both greater magnitude and greater distance.

64. From which, and from sect. 57 and 58, it is manifest that as we do not perceive the magnitudes of objects immediately by sight, so neither do we perceive them by the mediation of anything which has a necessary connexion with them. Those ideas that now suggest unto us the various magnitudes of external objects before we touch them, might possibly have suggested no such thing: or they might have signified them in a direct contrary manner: so that the very same ideas, on the perception whereof we judge an object to be small, might as well have served to make us conclude it great. Those ideas being in their own nature equally fitted to bring into our minds the idea of small or great, or no size at all of outward objects; just as the words of any language are in their own nature indifferent to signify this or that thing or nothing at all.

65. As we see distance, so we see magnitude. And we see both in the same way that we see shame or anger in the looks of a man. Those passions are themselves invisible, they are nevertheless let in by the eye along with colours and alterations of countenance, which are the immediate object of vision: and which signify them for no other reason than barely because they have been observed to accompany them. Without which

experience we should no more have taken blushing for a sign of shame than of gladness.

66. We are nevertheless exceeding prone to imagine those things which are perceived only by the mediation of others to be themselves the immediate objects of sight; or, at least, to have in their own nature a fitness to be suggested by them, before ever they had been experienced to coexist with them. From which prejudice everyone, perhaps, will not find it easy to emancipate himself, by any [but] the clearest convictions of reason. And there are some grounds to think that if there was one only invariable and universal languages in the world, and that men were born with the faculty of speaking it, it would be the opinion of many that the ideas of other men's minds were properly perceived by the ear, or had at least a necessary and inseparable tie with the sounds that were affixed to them. All which seems to arise from want of a due application of our discerning faculty, thereby to discriminate between the ideas that are in our understandings, and consider them apart from each other; which would preserve us from confounding those that are different, and make us see what ideas do, and what do not include or imply this or that other idea.

67. There is a celebrated phenomenon, the solution whereof I shall attempt to give by the principles that have been laid down, in reference to the manner wherein we apprehend by sight the magnitude of objects. The apparent magnitude of the moon when placed in the horizon is much greater than when it is in the meridian, though the angle under which the diameter of the moon is seen be not observed greater in the former case than in the latter: and the horizontal moon doth not constantly appear of the same bigness, but at some times seemeth far greater than at others.

68. Now in order to explain the reason of the moon's appearing greater than ordinary in the horizon, it must be observed that the particles which compose our atmosphere intercept the rays of light proceeding from any object to the eye; and by how much the greater is the portion of atmosphere interjacent between the object and the eye, by so much the more are the rays intercepted; and by consequence the appearance of the object rendered more faint, every object appearing more vigorous or more faint in proportion as it sendeth more or fewer rays into the eye. Now between the eye and the moon, when situated in the horizon, there lies a far greater quantity of atmosphere than there does when the moon is in the meridian. Whence it comes to pass that the appearance of the horizontal moon is fainter, and therefore by sect. 56 it should be thought bigger in that situation than in the meridian, or in any other elevation above the horizon.

69. Farther, the air being variously impregnated, sometimes more and sometimes less, with vapours and exhalations fitted to retund and intercept the rays of light, it follows that the appearance of the horizontal moon hath not always an equal faintness, and by consequence that luminary, though in the very same situation, is at one time judged greater than at another.

70. That we have here given the true account of the phenomena of the horizontal moon will, I suppose, be farther evident to anyone from the following considerations. FIRST, it is plain that which in this case suggests the idea of greater magnitude must be something which is itself perceived; for that which is unperceived cannot suggest to our perception any other thing. SECONDLY, it must be something that does not constantly remain the same, but is subject to some change or variation, since the appearance of the horizontal moon varies, being at one time greater than at another. And yet, THIRDLY, it cannot be the visible figure or magnitude, since that remains the same, or is rather lesser, by how much the moon is nearer to the horizon. It remains therefore that the true cause is that affection or alteration of the visible appearance which proceeds from the greater paucity of rays arriving at the eye, and which I term FAINTNESS: since this answers all the forementioned conditions, and I am not conscious of any other perception that doth.

71. Add to this that in misty weather it is a common observation that the appearance of the horizontal moon is far larger than usual, which greatly conspires with and strengthens our opinion. Neither would it prove in the least irreconcilable with what we have said, if the horizontal moon should chance sometimes to seem enlarged beyond its usual extent, even in more serene weather. For we must not only have regard to the mist which happens to be in the place where we stand; we ought also to take into our thoughts the whole sum of vapours and exhalations which lie betwixt the eye and the moon: all which cooperating to render the appearance of the moon more faint, and thereby increase its magnitude, it may chance to appear greater than it usually does, even in the horizontal position, at a time when, though there be no extraordinary fog or haziness, just in the place where we stand, yet the air between the eye and the moon, taken all together, may be loaded with a greater quantity of interspersed vapours and exhalations than at other times.

72. It may be objected that in consequence of our principles the interposition of a body in some degree opaque, which may intercept a great part of the rays of light, should render the appearance of the moon in the meridian as large as when it is viewed in the horizon.

To which I answer, it is not faintness anyhow applied that suggests greater magnitude, there being no necessary but only an experimental connexion between those two things. It follows that the faintness which enlarges the appearance must be applied in such sort, and with such circumstances, as have been observed to attend the vision of great magnitudes. When from a distance we behold great objects, the particles of the intermediate air and vapours, which are themselves unperceivable, do interrupt the rays of light, and thereby render the appearance less strong and vivid: now, faintness of appearance caused in this sort hath been experienced to coexist with great magnitude. But when it is caused by the interposition of an opaque sensible body, this circumstance alters the case, so that a faint appearance this way caused doth not suggest greater magnitude, because it hath not been experienced to coexist with it.

73. Faintness, as well as all other ideas or perceptions which suggest magnitude or distance, doth it in the same way that words suggest the notions to which they are annexed. Now, it is known a word pronounced with certain circumstances, or in a certain context with other words, hath not always the same import and signification that it hath when pronounced in some other circumstances or different context of words. The very same visible appearance as to faintness and all other respects, if placed on high, shall not suggest the same magnitude that it would if it were seen at an equal distance on a level with the eye. The reason whereof is that we are rarely accustomed to view objects at a great height; our concerns lie among things situated rather before than above us, and accordingly our eyes are not placed on the top of our heads, but in such a position as is most convenient for us to see distant objects standing in our way. And this situation of them being a circumstance which usually attends the vision of distant objects, we may from hence account for (what is commonly observed) an object's appearing of different magnitude, even with respect to its horizontal extension, on the top of a steeple, for example, an hundred feet high to one standing below, from what it would if placed at an hundred feet distance on a level with his eye. For it hath been shown that the judgment we make on the magnitude of a thing depends not on the visible appearance alone, but also on divers other circumstances, any one of which being omitted or varied may suffice to make some alteration in our judgment. Hence, the circumstances of viewing a distant object in such a situation as is usual, and suits with the ordinary posture of the head and eyes being omitted, and instead thereof a different situation of the object, which requires a different posture of the head taking place, it is not to be wondered at if the magnitude be judged different: but it will be demanded why an high object should constantly appear less than an equidistant low object of the same dimensions, for so it is observed to be: it

may indeed be granted that the variation of some circumstances may vary the judgment made on the magnitude of high objects, which we are less used to look at: but it does not hence appear why they should be judged less rather than greater? I answer that in case the magnitude of distant objects was suggested by the extent of their visible appearance alone, and thought proportional thereto, it is certain they would then be judged much less than now they seem to be (VIDE sect. 79). But several circumstances concurring to form the judgment we make on the magnitude of distant objects, by means of which they appear far larger than others, whose visible appearance hath an equal or even greater extension; it follows that upon the change or omission of any of those circumstances which are wont to attend the vision of distant objects, and so come to influence the judgments made on their magnitude, they shall proportionably appear less than otherwise they would. For any of those things that caused an object to be thought greater than in proportion to its visible extension being either omitted or applied without the usual circumstances, the judgment depends more entirely on the visible extension, and consequently the object must be judged less. Thus in the present case the situation of the thing seen being different from what it usually is in those objects we have occasion to view, and whose magnitude we observe, it follows that the very same object, being an hundred feet high, should seem less than if it was an hundred feet off on (or nearly on) a level with the eye. What has been here set forth seems to me to have no small share in contributing to magnify the appearance of the horizontal moon, and deserves not to be passed over in the explication of it.

74. If we attentively consider the phenomenon before us, we shall find the not discerning between the mediate and immediate objects of sight to be the chief cause of the difficulty that occurs in the explication of it. The magnitude of the visible moon, or that which is the proper and immediate object of vision, is not greater when the moon is in the horizon than when it is in the meridian. How comes it, therefore, to seem greater in one situation than the other? What is it can put this cheat on the understanding? It has no other perception of the moon than what it gets by sight: and that which is seen is of the same extent, I say, the visible appearance hath the same, or rather a less, magnitude when the moon is viewed in the horizontal than when in the meridional position: and yet it is esteemed greater in the former than in the latter. Herein consists the difficulty, which doth vanish and admit of a most easy solution, if we consider that as the visible moon is not greater in the horizon than in the meridian, so neither is it thought to be so. It hath been already shown that in any act of vision the visible object absolutely, or in itself, is little taken notice of, the mind still carrying its view from that to some tangible ideas

which have been observed to be connected with it, and by that means come to be suggested by it. So that when a thing is said to appear great or small, or whatever estimate be made of the magnitude of any thing, this is meant not of the visible but of the tangible object. This duly considered, it will be no hard matter to reconcile the seeming contradiction there is, that the moon should appear of a different bigness, the visible magnitude thereof remaining still the same. For by sect. 56 the very same visible extension, with a different faintness, shall suggest a different tangible extension. When therefore the horizontal moon is said to appear greater than the meridional moon, this must be understood not of a greater visible extension, but a of greater tangible or real extension, which by reason of the more than ordinary faintness of the visible appearance, is suggested to the mind along with it.

75. Many attempts have been made by learned men to account for this appearance. Gassendus, Descartes, Hobbes, and several others have employed their thoughts on that subject; but how fruitless and unsatisfactory their endeavours have been is sufficiently shown in THE TRANSACTIONS,[Phil. Trans. Num. 187. p. 314] where you may see their several opinions at large set forth and confuted, not without some surprize at the gross blunders that ingenious men have been forced into by endeavouring to reconcile this appearance with the ordinary Principles of optics. Since the writing of which there hath been published in the TRANSACTIONS [Numb. 187. P. 323] another paper relating to the same affair by the celebrated Dr. Wallis, wherein he attempts to account for that phenomenon which, though it seems not to contain anything new or different from what had been said before by others, I shall nevertheless consider in this place.

76. His opinion, in short, is this; we judge not of the magnitude of an object by the visual angle alone, but by the visual angle in conjunction with the distance. Hence, though the angle remain the same, or even become less, yet if withal the distance seem to have been increased, the object shall appear greater. Now, one way whereby we estimate the distance of anything is by the number and extent of the intermediate objects: when therefore the moon is seen in the horizon, the variety of fields, houses, etc., together with the large prospect of the wide extended land or sea that lies between the eye and the utmost limb of the horizon, suggest unto the mind the idea of greater distance, and consequently magnify the appearance. And this, according to Dr. Wallis, is the true account of the extraordinary largeness attributed by the mind to the horizontal moon at a time when the angle subtended by its diameter is not one jot greater than it used to be.

77. With reference to this opinion, not to repeat what hath been already said concerning distance, I shall only observe, FIRST, that if the prospect of interjacent objects be that which suggests the idea of farther distance, and this idea of farther distance be the cause that brings into the mind the idea of greater magnitude, it should hence follow that if one looked at the horizontal moon from behind a wall, it would appear no bigger than ordinary. For in that case the wall interposing cuts off all that prospect of sea and land, etc. which might otherwise increase the apparent distance, and thereby the apparent magnitude of the moon. Nor will it suffice to say the memory doth even then suggest all that extent of land, etc., which lies within the horizon; which suggestion occasions a sudden judgment of sense that the moon is farther off and larger than usual. For ask any man who, from such a station beholding the horizontal moon, shall think her greater than usual, whether he hath at that time in his mind any idea of the intermediate objects, or long tract of land that lies between his eye and the extreme edge of the horizon? And whether it be that idea which is the cause of his making the aforementioned judgment? He will, I suppose, reply in the negative, and declare the horizontal moon shall appear greater than the meridional, though he never thinks of all or any of those things that lie between him and it. SECONDLY, it seems impossible by this hypothesis to account for the moon's appearing in the very same situation at one time greater than at another; which nevertheless has been shown to be very agreeable to the principles we have laid down, and receives a most easy and natural explication from them. For the further clearing' up of this point it is to be observed that what we immediately and properly see are only lights and colours in sundry situations and shades and degrees of faintness and clearness, confusion and distinctness. All which visible objects are only in the mind, nor do they suggest ought external, whether distance or magnitude, otherwise than by habitual connexion as words do things. We are also to remark that, beside the straining of the eyes, and beside the vivid and faint, the distinct and confused appearances (which, bearing some proportion to lines and angles, have been substituted instead of them in the foregoing part of this treatise), there are other means which suggest both distance and magnitude; particularly the situation of visible points of objects, as upper or lower; the one suggesting a farther distance and greater magnitude, the other a nearer distance and lesser magnitude: all which is an effect only of custom and experience; there being really nothing intermediate in the line of distance between the uppermost and lowermost, which are both equidistant, or rather at no distance from the eye, as there is also nothing in upper or lower, which by necessary connexion should suggest greater or lesser magnitude. Now, as these customary, experimental means of suggesting distance do likewise suggest magnitude, so they suggest the one as immediately as the other. I say

they do not (VIDE sect. 53) first suggest distance, and then leave the mind from thence to infer or compute magnitude, jut suggest magnitude as immediately and directly as they suggest distance.

78. This phenomenon of the horizontal moon is a clear instance of the insufficiency of lines and angles for explaining the way wherein the mind perceives and estimates the magnitude of outward objects. There is nevertheless a use of computation by them in order to determine the apparent magnitude of things, so far as they have a connexion with, and are proportional to, those other ideas or perceptions which are the true and immediate occasions that suggest to the mind the apparent magnitude of things. But this in general may, I think, be observed concerning mathematical computation in optics: that it can never be very precise and exact since the judgments we make of the magnitude of external things do often depend on several circumstances, which are not proportionable to, or capable of being defined by, lines and angles.

79. From what has been said we may safely deduce this consequence; to wit, that a man born blind and made to see would, at first opening of his eyes, make a very different judgment of the magnitude of objects intromitted by them from what others do. He would not consider the ideas of sight with reference to, or as having any connexion with, the ideas of touch: his view of them being entirely terminated within themselves, he can no otherwise judge them great or small than as they contain a greater or lesser number of visible points. Now, it being certain that any visible point can cover or exclude from view only one other visible point, it follows that whatever object intercepts the view of another hath an equal number of visible points with it; and consequently they shall both be thought by him to have the same magnitude. Hence it is evident one in those circumstances would judge his thumb, with which he might hide a tower or hinder its being seen, equal to that tower, or his hand, the interposition whereof might conceal experimental means the firmament from his view, equal to the firmament: how great an inequality soever there may in our apprehensions seem to be betwixt those two things, because of the customary and close connexion that has grown up in our minds between the objects of sight and touch; whereby the very different and distinct ideas of those two senses are so blended and confounded together as to be mistaken for one and the same thing; out of which prejudice we cannot easily extricate ourselves.

80. For the better explaining the nature of vision, and setting the manner wherein we perceive magnitudes in a due light, I shall proceed to make some observations concerning

matters relating thereto, whereof the want of reflexion, and duly separating between tangible and visible ideas, is apt to create in us mistaken and confused notions. And FIRST, I shall observe that the MINIMUM VISIBILE is exactly equal in all beings whatsoever that are endowed with the visive faculty. No exquisite formation of the eye, no peculiar sharpness of sight, can make it less in one creature than in another; for it not being distinguishable into parts, nor in any wise a consisting of them, it must necessarily be the same to all. For suppose it otherwise, and that the MINIMUM VISIBILE of a mite, for instance, be less than the MINIMUM VISIBILE of a man: the latter therefore may by detraction of some part be made equal to the former: it doth therefore consist of parts, which is inconsistent with the notion of a MINIMUM VISIBILE or point.

81. It will perhaps be objected that the MINIMUM VISIBILE of a man doth really and in itself contain parts whereby it surpasses that of a mite, though they are not perceivable by the man. To which I answer, the MINIMUM VISIBILE having (in like manner as all other the proper and immediate objects of sight) been shown not to have any existence without the mind of him who sees it, it follows there cannot be any pan of it that is not actually perceived, and therefore visible. Now for any object to contain distinct visible parts, and at the same time to be a MINIMUM VISIBILE, is a manifest contradiction.

82. Of these visible points we see at all times an equal number. It is every whit as great when our view is contracted and bounded by near objects as when it is extended to larger and remoter. For it being impossible that one MINIMUM VISIBILE should obscure or keep out of sight mote than one other, it is a plain consequence that when my view is on all sides bounded by the walls of my study see just as many visible points as I could, in case that by the removal of the study–walls and all other obstructions, I had a full prospect of the circumjacent fields, mountains, sea, and open firmament: for so long as I am shut up within the walls, by their interposition every point of the external objects is covered from my view: but each point that is seen being able to cover or exclude from sight one only other corresponding point, it follows that whilst my sight is confined to those narrow walls I see as many points, or MINIMA VISIBILIA, as I should were those walls away, by looking on all the external objects whose prospect is intercepted by them. Whenever therefore we are said to have a greater prospect at one time than another, this must be understood with relation, not to the proper and immediate, but the secondary and mediate objects of vision, which, as hath been shown, properly belong to the touch.

83. The visive faculty considered with reference to its immediate objects may be found to labour of two defects. FIRST, in respect of the extent or number of visible points that are at once perceivable by it, which is narrow and limited to a certain degree. It can take in at one view but a certain determinate number of MINIMA VISIBILIA, beyond which it cannot extend its prospect. Secondly, our sight is defective in that its view is not only narrow, but also for the most part confused: of those things that we take in at one prospect we can see but a few at once clearly and unconfusedly: and the more we fix our sight on any one object, by so much the darker and more indistinct shall the rest appear.

84. Corresponding to these two defects of sight, we may imagine as many perfections, to wit, 1ST, that of comprehending in one view a greater number of visible points. 2DLY, of being able to view them all equally and at once with the utmost clearness and distinction. That those perfections are not actually in some intelligences of a different order and capacity from ours it is impossible for us to know.

85. In neither of those two ways do microscopes contribute to the improvement of sight; for when we look through a microscope we neither see more visible points, nor are the collateral points more distinct than when we look with the naked eye at objects placed in a due distance. A microscope brings us, as it were, into a new world: it presents us with a new scene of visible objects quite different from what we behold with the naked eye. But herein consists the most remarkable difference, to wit, that whereas the objects perceived by the eye alone have a certain connexion with tangible objects, whereby we are taught to foresee what will ensue upon the approach or application of distant objects to the parts of our own body, which much conduceth to its preservation, there is not the like connexion between things tangible and those visible objects that are perceived by help of a fine microscope.

86. Hence it is evident that were our eyes turned into the nature of microscopes, we should not be much benefited by the change; we should be deprived of the forementioned advantage we at present receive by the visive faculty, and have left us only the empty amusement of seeing, without any other benefit arising from it. But in that case, it will perhaps be said, our sight would be endued with a far greater sharpness and penetration than it now hath. But it is certain from what we have already shown that the MINIMUM VISIBILE is never greater or lesser, but in all cases constantly the same: and in the case of microscopical eyes I see only this difference, to wit, that upon the ceasing of a certain observable connexion betwixt the divers perceptions of sight and touch, which before

enabled us to regulate our actions by the eye, it would now be rendered utterly unserviceable to that purpose.

87. Upon the whole it seems that if we consider the use and end of sight, together with the present state and circumstances of our being, we shall not find any great cause to complain of any defect or imperfection in it, or easily conceive how it could be mended. With such admirable wisdom is that faculty contrived, both for the pleasure and convenience of life.

88. Having finished what I intended to say concerning the distance and magnitude of objects, I come now to treat of the manner wherein the mind perceives by sight their situation. Among the discoveries of the last age, it is reputed none of the least that the manner of vision hath been more clearly explained than ever it had been before. There is at this day no one ignorant that the pictures of external objects are painted on the RETINA, or fund of the eye: that we can see nothing which is not so painted: and that, according as the picture is more distinct or confused, so also is the perception we have of the object: but then in this explication of vision there occurs one mighty difficulty. The objects are painted in an inverted order on the bottom of the eye: the upper part of any object being painted on the lower part of the eye, and the lower part of the object on the upper part of the eye: and so also as to right and left. Since therefore the pictures are thus inverted, it is demanded how it comes to pass that we see the objects erect and in their natural posture?

89. In answer to this difficulty we are told that the mind, perceiving an impulse of a ray of light on the upper part of the eye, considers this ray as coming in a direct line from the lower part of the object; and in like manner tracing the ray that strikes on the lower part of the eye, it is directed to the upper part of the object. Thus in the adjacent figure, C, the lower point of the object ABC, is projected on C the upper part of the eye. So likewise the highest point A is projected on A the lowest part of the eye, which makes the representation CBA inverted: but the mind considering the stroke that is made on C as coming in the straight line CC from the lower end of the object; and the stroke or impulse on a as coming in the line AA from the upper end of the object, is directed to make a right judgment of the situation of the object ABC, notwithstanding the picture of it is inverted. This is illustrated by conceiving a blind man who, holding in his hands two sticks that cross each other, doth with them touch the extremities of an object, placed in a perpendicular situation. It is certain this man will judge that to be the upper part of the

30

object which he touches with the stick held in the undermost hand, and that to be the lower part of the object which he touches with the stick in his uppermost hand. This is the common explication of the erect appearance of objects, which is generally received and acquiesced in, being (as Mr. Molyneux tells us [Diopt. par. 2. c. 7. P. 289.]) 'allowed by all men as satisfactory'.

90. But this account to me does not seem in any degree true. Did I perceive those impulses, decussations, and directions of the rays of light in like manner as hath been set forth, then indeed it would not be altogether void of probability. And there might be some pretence for the comparison of the blind man and his cross sticks. But the case is far otherwise. I know very well that I perceive no such thing. And of consequence I cannot thereby make an estimate of the situation of objects. I appeal to anyone's experience, whether he be conscious to himself that he thinks on the intersection made by the radious [SIC] pencils, or pursues the impulses they give in right lines, whenever he perceives by sight the position of any object? To me it seems evident that crossing and tracing of the rays is never thought on by children, idiots, or in truth by any other, save only those who have applied themselves to the study of optics. And for the mind to judge of the situation of objects by those things without perceiving them, or to perceive them without knowing it, is equally beyond my comprehension. Add to this that the explaining the manner of vision by the example of cross sticks and hunting for the object along the axes of the radious pencils, doth suppose the proper objects of sight to be perceived at a distance from us, contrary to what hath been demonstrated.

91. It remains, therefore, that we look for some other explication of this difficulty: and I believe it not impossible to find one, provided we examine it to the bottom, and carefully distinguish between the ideas of sight and touch; which cannot be too oft inculcated in treating of vision: but more especially throughout the consideration of this affair we ought to carry that distinction in our thoughts: for that from want of a right understanding thereof the difficulty of explaining erect vision seems chiefly to arise.

92. In order to disentangle our minds from whatever prejudices we may entertain with relation to the subject in hand, nothing seems more apposite than the taking into our thoughts the case of one born blind, and afterwards, when grown up, made to see. And though, perhaps, it may not be an easy task to divest ourselves entirely of the experience received from sight, so as to be able to put our thoughts exactly in the posture of such a one's, we must, nevertheless, as far as possible, endeavour to frame true conceptions of

what might reasonably be supposed to pass in his mind.

93. It is certain that a man actually blind, and who had continued so from his birth, would by the sense of feeling attain to have ideas of upper and lower. By the motion of his hand he might discern the situation of any tangible object placed within his FI reach. That part on which he felt himself supported, or towards which he perceived his body to gravitate, he would term lower, and the contrary to this upper; and accordingly denominate whatsoever objects he touched.

94. But then, whatever judgments he makes concerning the situation of objects are confined to those only that are perceivable by touch. All those things that are intangible and of a spiritual nature, his thoughts and desires, his passions, and in general all the modifications of the soul, to these he would never apply the terms UPPER and LOWER, except only in a metaphorical sense. He may, perhaps, by way of allusion, speak of high or low thoughts: but those terms in their proper signification would never be applied to anything that was not conceived to exist without the mind. For a man born blind, and remaining in the same state, could mean nothing else by the words HIGHER and LOWER than a greater or lesser distance from the earth; which distance he would measure by the motion or application of his hand or some other part of his body. It is therefore evident that all those things which, in respect of each other, would by him be thought higher or lower, must be such as were conceived to exist without his mind, in the ambient space.

95. Whence it plainly follows that such a one, if we suppose him made to see, would not at first sight think anything he saw was high or low, erect or inverted; for it hath been already demonstrated in sect. 41 that he would not think the things he perceived by sight to be at any distance from him, or without his mind. The objects to which he had hitherto been used to apply the terms UP and DOWN, HIGH and LOW, were such only as affected or were some way perceived by his couch: but the proper objects of vision make a new set of ideas, perfectly distinct and different from the former, and which can in no sort make themselves perceived by touch. There is, therefore, nothing at all that could induce him to think those terms applicable to them: nor would he ever think it till such time as he had observed their connexion with tangible objects, and the same prejudice began to insinuate itself into his understanding, which from their infancy had grown up in the understandings of other men.

96. To set this matter in a clearer light I shall make use of an example. Suppose the above–mentioned blind person by his touch perceives a man to stand erect. Let us inquire into the manner of this. By the application of his hand to the several parts of a human body he had perceived different tangible ideas, which being collected into sundry complex ones, have distinct names annexed to them. Thus one combination of a certain tangible figure, bulk, and consistency of parts is called the head, another the hand, a third the foot, and so of the rest: all which complex ideas could, in his understanding, be made up only of ideas perceivable by touch. He had also by his touch obtained an idea of earth or ground, towards which he perceives the parts of his body to have a natural tendency. Now, by ERECT nothing more being meant than that perpendicular position of a man wherein his feet are nearest to the earth, if the blind person by moving his hand over the parts of the man who stands before him perceives the tangible ideas that compose the head to be farthest from, and those that compose the feet to be nearest to, that other combination of tangible ideas which he calls earth, he will denominate that man erect. But if we suppose him on a sudden to receive his sight, and that he behold a man standing before him, it is evident in that case he would neither judge the man he sees to be erect nor inverted; for he never having known those terms applied to any other save tangible things, or which existed in the space without him, and what he sees neither being tangible nor perceived as existing without, he could not know that in propriety of language they were applicable to it.

97. Afterwards, when upon turning his head or eyes up and down to the right and left he shall observe the visible objects to change, and shall also attain to know that they are called by the same names, and connected with the objects perceived by touch; then indeed he will come to speak of them and their situation, in the same terms that he has been used to apply to tangible things; and those that he perceives by turning up his eyes he will call upper, and those that by turning down his eyes he will call lower.

98. And this seems to me the true reason why he should think those objects uppermost that are painted on the lower part of his eye: for by turning the eye up they shall be distinctly seen; as likewise those that are painted on the highest part of the eye shall be distinctly seen by turning the eye down, and are for that reason esteemed lowest; for we have shown that to the immediate objects of sight considered in themselves, he would not attribute the terms HIGH and LOW. It must therefore be on account of some circumstances which are observed to attend them: and these, it is plain, are the actions of turning the eye up and down, which suggest a very obvious reason why the mind should

denominate the objects of sight accordingly high or low. And without this motion of the eye, this turning it up and down in order to discern different objects, doubtless ERECT, INVERSE, and other the like terms relating to the position of tangible objects, would never have been transferred, or in any degree apprehended to belong to the ideas of sight: the mere act of seeing including nothing in it to that purpose; whereas the different situations of the eye naturally direct the mind to make a suitable judgment of the situation of objects intromitted by it.

99. Farther, when he has by experience learned the connexion there is between the several ideas of sight and touch, he will be able, by the perception he has of the situation of visible things in respect of one another, to make a sudden and true estimate of the situation of outward, tangible things corresponding to them. And thus it is he shall perceive by sight the situation of external objects which do not properly fall under that sense.

100. I know we are very prone to think that, if just made to see, we should judge of the situation of visible things as we do now: but we are also as prone to think that, at first sight, we should in the same way apprehend the distance and magnitude of objects as we do now: which hath been shown to be a false and groundless persuasion. And for the like reasons the same censure may be passed on the positive assurance that most men, before they have thought sufficiently of the matter, might have of their being able to determine by the eye at first view, whether objects were erect or inverse.

101. It will, perhaps, be objected co our opinion that a man, for instance, being thought erect when his feet are next the earth, and inverted when his head is next the earth, it doth hence follow that by the mere act of vision, without any experience or altering the situation of the eye, we should have determined whether he were erect or inverted: for both the earth itself, and the limbs of the man who stands thereon, being equally perceived by sight, one cannot choose seeing what part of the man is nearest the earth, and what part farthest from it, i.e. whether he be erect or inverted.

102. To which I answer, the ideas which constitute the tangible earth and man are entirely different from those which constitute the visible earth and man. Nor was it possible, by virtue of the visive faculty alone, without superadding any experience of touch, or altering the position of the eye, ever to have known, or so much as suspected, there had been any relation or connexion between them. Hence a man at first view would not

denominate anything he saw earth, or head, or foot; and consequently he could not tell by the mere act of vision whether the head or feet were nearest the earth: nor, indeed, would we have thereby any thought of earth or man, erect or inverse, at all: which will be made yet more evident if we nicely observe, and make a particular comparison between, the ideas of both senses.

103. That which I see is only variety of light and colours. That which I feel is hard or soft, hot or cold, rough or smooth. What similitude, what connexion have those ideas with these? Or how is it possible that anyone should see reason to give one and the same name to combinations of ideas so very different before he had experienced their coexistence? We do not find there is any necessary connexion betwixt this or that tangible quality and any colour whatsoever. And we may sometimes perceive colours where there is nothing to be felt. All which doth make it manifest that no man, at first receiving of his sight, would know there was any agreement between this or that particular object of his sight and any object of touch he had been already acquainted with: the colours, therefore, of the head would to him no more suggest the idea of head than they would the idea of foot.

104. Farther, we have at large shown (VID. sect. 63 and 64) there is no discoverable necessary connexion between any given visible magnitude and any one particular tangible magnitude; but that it is entirely the result of custom and experience, and depends on foreign and accidental circumstances that we can by the perception of visible extension inform ourselves what may be the extension of any tangible object connected with it. Hence it is certain that neither the visible magnitude of head or foot would bring along with them into the mind, at first opening of the eyes, the respective tangible magnitudes of those parts.

105. By the foregoing section it is plain the visible figure of any part of the body hath no necessary connexion with the tangible figure thereof, so as at first sight to suggest it to the mind. For figure is the termination of magnitude; whence it follows that no visible magnitude having in its own nature an aptness to suggest any one particular tangible magnitude, so neither can any visible figure be inseparably connected with its corresponding tangible figure: so as of itself and in a way prior to experience, it might suggest it to the understanding. This will be farther evident if we consider that what seems smooth and round to the touch may to sight, if viewed through a microscope, seem quite otherwise.

106. From all which laid together and duly considered, we may clearly deduce this inference. In the first act of vision no idea entering by the eye would have a perceivable connexion with the ideas to which the names EARTH, MAN, HEAD, FOOT, etc., were annexed in the understanding of a person blind from his birth; so as in any sort to introduce them into his mind, or make themselves be called by the same names, and reputed the same things with them, as afterwards they come to be.

107. There doth, nevertheless, remain one difficulty, which perhaps may seem to press hard on our opinion, and deserve not to be passed over: for though it be granted that neither the colour, size, nor figure of the visible feet have any necessary connexion with the ideas that compose the tangible feet, so as to bring them at first sight into my mind, or make me in danger of confounding them before I had been used to, and for some time experienced their connexion: yet thus much seems undeniable, namely, that the number of the visible feet being the same with that of the tangible feet, I may from hence without any experience of sight reasonably conclude that they represent or are connected with the feet rather than the head. I say, it seems the idea of two visible feet will sooner suggest to the mind the idea of two tangible feet than of one head; so that the blind man upon first reception of the visive faculty might know which were the feet or two, and which the head or one.

108. In order to get clear of this seeming difficulty we need only observe that diversity of visible objects doth not necessarily infer diversity of tangible objects corresponding to them. A picture painted with great variety of colours affects the touch in one uniform manner; it is therefore evident that I do not by any necessary consecution, independent of experience, judge of the number of things tangible from the number of things visible. I should not, therefore, at first opening my eyes conclude that because I see two I shall feel two. How, therefore, can I, before experience teaches me, know that the visible legs, because two, are connected with the tangible legs, or the visible head, because one, is connected with the tangible head? The truth is, the things I see are so very different and heterogeneous from the things I feel that the perception of the one would never have suggested the other to my thoughts, or enabled me to pass the least judgment thereon, until I had experienced their connexion.

109. But for a fuller illustration of this matter it ought to be considered that number (however some may reckon it amongst the primary qualities) is nothing fixed and settled, really existing in things themselves. It is entirely the creature of the mind, considering

either an idea by itself, or any combination of ideas to which it gives one name, and so makes it pass for an unit. According as the mind variously combines its ideas the unit varies: and as the unit, so the number, which is only a collection of units, doth also vary. We call a window one, a chimney one, and yet a house in which there are many windows and many chimneys hath an equal right to be called one, and many houses go to the making of the city. In these and the like, instances it is evident the unit constantly relates to the particular draughts the mind makes of its ideas, to which it affixes names, and wherein it includes more or less as best suits its own ends and purposes. Whatever, therefore, the mind considers as one, that is an unit. Every combination of ideas is considered as one thing by the mind, and in token thereof is marked by one name. Now, this naming and combining together of ideas is perfectly arbitrary, and done by the mind in such sort as experience shows it to be most convenient: without which our ideas had never been collected into such sundry distinct combinations as they now are.

110. Hence it follows that a man born blind and afterwards, when grown up, made to see, would not in the first act of vision parcel out the ideas of sight into the same distinct collections that others do, who have experienced which do regularly coexist and are proper to be bundled up together under one name. He would not, for example, make into one complex idea, and thereby esteem an unit, all those particular ideas which constitute the visible head or foot. For there can be no reason assigned why he should do so, barely upon his seeing a man stand upright before him. There crowd into his mind the ideas which compose the visible man, in company with all the other ideas of sight perceived at the same time: but all these ideas offered at once to his view, he would not distribute into sundry distinct combinations till such time as by observing the motion of the parts of the man and other experiences he comes to know which are to be separated and which to be collected together.

111. From what hath been premised it is plain the objects of sight and touch make, if I may so say, two sets of ideas which are widely different from each other. To objects of either kind we indifferently attribute the terms high and low, right and left, and suchlike, denoting the position or situation of things: but then we must well observe that the position of any object is determined with respect only to objects of the same sense. We say any object of touch is high or low, according as it is more or less distant from the tangible earth: and in like manner we denominate any object of sight high or low in proportion as it is more or less distant from the visible earth: but to define the situation of visible things with relation to the distance they bear from any tangible thing, or VICE

VERSA, this were absurd and perfectly unintelligible. For all visible things are equally in the mind, and take up no part of the external space: and consequently are equidistant from any tangible thing which exists without the mind.

112. Or rather, to speak truly, the proper objects of sight are at no distance, neither near nor far, from any tangible thing. For if we inquire narrowly into the matter we shall find that those things only are compared together in respect of distance which exist after the same manner, or appertain unto the same sense. For by the distance between any two points nothing more is meant than the number of intermediate points: if the given points are visible the distance between them is marked out by the number of the interjacent visible points: if they are tangible, the distance between them is a line consisting of tangible points; but if they are one tangible and the other visible, the distance between them doth neither consist of points perceivable by sight nor by touch, i.e. it is utterly inconceivable. This, perhaps, will not find an easy admission into all men's understanding: however, I should gladly be informed whether it be not true by anyone who will be at the pains to reflect a little and apply it home to his thoughts.

113. The not observing what has been delivered in the two last sections seems to have occasioned no small part of the difficulty that occurs in the business of erect appearances. The head, which is painted nearest the earth, seems to be farthest from it: and on the other hand the feet, which are painted farthest from the earth, are thought nearest to it. Herein lies the difficulty, which vanishes if we express the thing more clearly and free from ambiguity, thus: how comes it that to the eye the visible head which is nearest the tangible earth seems farthest from the earth, and the visible feet, which are farthest from the tangible earth seem nearest the earth? The question being thus proposed, who sees not the difficulty is founded on a supposition that the eye, or visive faculty, or rather the soul by means thereof, should judge of the situation of visible objects with reference to their distance from the tangible earth? Whereas it is evident the tangible earth is not perceived by sight: and it hath been shown in the two last preceding sections that the location of visible objects is determined only by the distance they bear from one another; and that it is nonsense to talk of distance, far or near, between a visible and tangible thing.

114. If we confine our thoughts to the proper objects of sight, the whole is plain and easy. The head is painted farthest from, and the feet nearest to, the visible earth; and so they appear to be. What is there strange or unaccountable in this? Let us suppose the pictures in the fund of the eye to be the immediate objects of the sight. The consequence is that

things should appear in the same posture they are painted in; and is it not so? The head which is seen seems farthest from the earth which is seen; and the feet which are seen seem nearest to the earth, which is seen; and just so they are painted.

115. But, say you, the picture of the man is inverted, and yet the appearance is erect: I ask, what mean you by the picture of the man, or, which is the same thing, the visible man's being inverted? You tell me it is inverted, because the heels are uppermost and the head undermost? Explain me this. You say that by the head's being undermost you mean that it is nearest to the earth; and by the heels being uppermost that they are farthest from the earth. I ask again what earth you mean? You cannot mean the earth that is painted on the eye, or the visible earth: for the picture of the head is farthest from the picture of the earth, and the picture of the feet nearest to the picture of the earth; and accordingly the visible head is farthest from the visible earth, and the visible feet nearest to it. It remains, therefore, that you mean the tangible earth, and so determine the situation of visible things with respect to tangible things; contrary to what hath been demonstrated in sect. 111 and 112. The two distinct provinces of sight and touch should be considered apart, and as if their objects had no intercourse, no manner of relation one to another, in point of distance or position.

116. Farther, what greatly contributes to make us mistake in this matter is that when we think of the pictures in the fund of the eye, we imagine ourselves looking on the fund of another's eye, or another looking on the fund of our own eye, and beholding the pictures painted thereon. Suppose two eyes A and B: A from some distance looking on the pictures in B sees them inverted, and for that reason concludes they are inverted in B: but this is wrong. There are projected in little on the bottom of A the images of the pictures of, suppose, man, earth, etc., which are painted on B. And besides these the eye B itself, and the objects which environ it, together with another earth, are projected in a larger size on A. Now, by the eye A these larger images are deemed the true objects, and the lesser only pictures in miniature. And it is with respect to those greater images that it determines the situation of the smaller images: so that comparing the little man with the great earth, A judges him inverted, or that the feet are farthest from and the head nearest to the great earth. Whereas, if A compare the little man with the little earth, then he will appear erect, i.e. his head shall seem farthest from, and his feet nearest to, the little earth. But we must consider that B does not see two earths as A does: it sees only what is represented by the little pictures in A, and consequently shall judge the man erect. For, in truth, the man in B is not inverted, for there the feet are next the earth; but it is the

representation of it in A which is inverted, for there the head of the representation of the picture of the man in B is next the earth, and the feet farthest from the earth, meaning the earth which is without the representation of the pictures in B. For if you take the little images of the pictures in B, and consider them by themselves, and with respect only to one another, they are all erect and in their natural posture.

117. Farther, there lies a mistake in our imagining that the pictures of external objects are painted on the bottom of the eye. It hath been shown there is no resemblance BETWEEN the ideas of sight and things tangible. It hath likewise been demonstrated that the proper objects of sight do not exist without the mind. Whence it clearly follows that the pictures painted on the bottom of the eye are not the pictures of external objects. Let anyone consult his own thoughts, and then say what affinity, what likeness there is between that certain variety and disposition of colours which constitute the visible man, or picture of a man, and that other combination of far different ideas, sensible by touch, which compose the tangible man. But if this be the case, how come they to be accounted pictures or images, since that supposes them to copy or represent some originals or other?

118. To which I answer: in the forementioned instance the eye A takes the little images, included within the representation of the other eye B, to be pictures or copies, whereof the archetypes are not things existing without, but the larger pictures projected on its own fund: and which by A are not thought pictures, but the originals, or true things themselves. Though if we suppose a third eye C from a due distance to behold the fund of A, then indeed the things projected thereon shall, to C, seem pictures or images in the same sense that those projected on B do to A.

119. Rightly to conceive this point we must carefully distinguish between the ideas of sight and touch, between the visible and tangible eye; for certainly on the tangible eye nothing either is or seems to be painted. Again, the visible eye, as well as all other visible objects, hath been shown to exist only in the mind, which perceiving its own ideas, and comparing them together, calls some PICTURES in respect of others. What hath been said, being rightly comprehended and laid together, doth, I think, afford a full and genuine explication of the erect appearance of objects; which phenomenon, I must confess, I do not see how it can be explained by any theories of vision hitherto made public.

120. In treating of these things the use of language is apt to occasion some obscurity and confusion, and create in us wrong ideas; for language being accommodated to the common notions and prejudices of men, it is scarce possible to deliver the naked and precise truth without great circumlocution, impropriety, and (to an unwary reader) seeming contradictions; I do therefore once for all desire whoever shall think it worth his while to understand what I have written concerning vision, that he would not stick in this or that phrase, or manner of expression, but candidly collect my meaning from the whole sum and tenor of my discourse, and laying aside the words as much as possible, consider the bare notions themselves, and then judge whether they are agreeable to truth and his own experience, or no.

121. We have shown the way wherein the mind by mediation of visible ideas doth perceive or apprehend the distance, magnitude and situation of tangible objects. We come now to inquire more particularly concerning the difference between the ideas of sight and touch, which are called by the same names, and see whether there be any idea common to both senses. From what we have at large set forth and demonstrated in the foregoing parts of this treatise, it is plain there is no one selfsame numerical extension perceived both by sight and touch; but that the particular figures and extensions perceived by sight, however they may be called by the same names and reputed the same things with those perceived by touch, are nevertheless different, and have an existence distinct and separate from them: so that the question is not now concerning the same numerical ideas, but whether there be any one and the same sort of species of ideas equally perceivable to both senses; or, in other words, whether extension, figure, and motion perceived by sight are not specifically distinct from extension, figure, and motion perceived by touch.

122. But before I come more particularly to discuss this matter, I find it proper to consider extension in abstract: for of this there is much talk, and I am apt to think that when men speak of extension as being an idea common to two senses, it is with a secret supposition that we can single out extension from all other tangible and visible qualities, and form thereof an abstract idea, which idea they will have common both to sight and touch. We are therefore to understand by extension in abstract an idea of extension, for instance, a line or surface entirely stripped of all other sensible qualities and circumstances that might determine it to any particular existence; it is neither black nor white, nor red, nor hath it any colour at all, or any tangible quality whatsoever and consequently it is of no finite determinate magnitude: for that which bounds or distinguishes one extension from another is some quality or circumstance wherein they

disagree.

123. Now I do not find that I can perceive, imagine, or any wise frame in my mind such an abstract idea as is here spoken of. A line or surface which is neither black, nor white, nor blue, nor yellow, etc., nor long, nor short, nor rough, nor smooth, nor square, nor round, etc., is perfectly incomprehensible. This I am sure of as to myself: how far the faculties of other men may reach they best can tell.

124. It is commonly said that the object of geometry is abstract extension: but geometry contemplates figures: now, figure is the termination of magnitude: but we have shown that extension in abstract hath no finite determinate magnitude. Whence it clearly follows that it can have no figure, and consequently is not the object of geometry. It is indeed a tenet as well of the modern as of the ancient philosophers that all general truths are concerning universal abstract ideas; without which, we are told, there could be no science, no demonstration of any general proposition in geometry. But it were no hard matter, did I think it necessary to my present purpose, to show that propositions and demonstrations in geometry might be universal, though they who make them never think of abstract general ideas of triangles or circles.

125. After reiterated endeavours to apprehend the general idea a triangle, I have found it altogether incomprehensible. And surely if anyone were able to introduce that idea into my mind, it must be the author of the ESSAY CONCERNING HUMAN UNDERSTANDING; he who has so far distinguished himself from the generality of writers by the clearness and significancy of what he says. Let us therefore see how this celebrated author describes the general or abstract idea of a triangle. 'It must be (says he) neither oblique nor rectangular, neither equilateral, equicrural, nor scalenum; but all and none of these at once. In effect, it is somewhat imperfect that cannot exist; an idea, wherein some parts of several different and inconsistent ideas are put together' ESSAY ON HUM. UNDERSTAND. B. iv. C. 7. S.9. This is the idea which he thinks needful for the enlargement of knowledge, which is the subject of mathematical demonstration, and without which we could never come to know any general proposition concerning triangles. That author acknowledges it doth 'require some pains and skill to form this general idea of a triangle.' IBID. But had he called to mind what he says in another place, to wit, 'That ideas of mixed modes wherein any inconsistent ideas are put together cannot so much as exist in the mind, i.e. be conceived.' VID. B. iii. C. 10. S. 33. IBID. I say, had this occurred to his thoughts, it is not improbable he would have owned it above all the

pains and skill he was master of to form the above-mentioned idea of a triangle, which is made up of manifest, staring contradictions. That a man who laid so great a stress on clear and determinate ideas should nevertheless talk at this rate seems very surprising. But the wonder will lessen if it be considered that the source whence this opinion flows is the prolific womb which has brought forth innumerable errors and difficulties in all parts of philosophy and in all the sciences: but this matter, taken in its full extent, were a subject too comprehensive to be insisted on in this place. And so much for extension in abstract.

126. Some, perhaps, may think pure space, VACUUM, or trine dimension to be equally the object of sight and touch: but though we have a very great propension to think the ideas of outness and space to be the immediate object of sight, yet, if I mistake not, in the foregoing parts of this essay that hath been clearly demonstated to be a mere delusion, arising from the quick and sudden suggestion of fancy, which so closely connects the idea of distance with those of sight, that we are apt to think it is itself a proper and immediate object of that sense till reason corrects the mistake.

127. It having been shown that there are no abstract ideas of figure, and that it is impossible for us by any precision of thought to frame an idea of extension separate from all other visible and tangible qualities which shall be common both to sight and touch: the question now remaining is, whether the particular extensions, figures, and motions perceived by sight be of the same kind with the particular extensions, figures, and motions perceived by touch? In answer to which I shall venture to lay down the following proposition: THE EXTENSION, FIGURES, AND MOTIONS PERCEIVED BY SIGHT ARE SPECIFICALLY DISTINCT FROM THE IDEAS OF TOUCH CALLED BY THE SAME NAMES, NOR is THERE ANY SUCH THING as ONE IDEA OR KIND OF IDEA COMMON TO BOTH SENSES. This proposition may without much difficulty be collected from what hath been said in several places of this essay. But because it seems so remote from, and contrary to, the received notions and settled opinion of mankind, I shall attempt to demonstrate it more particularly and at large by the following arguments.

128. When upon perception of an idea I range it under this or that sort, it is because it is perceived after the same manner, or because it has a likeness or conformity with, or affects me in the same way as, the ideas of the sort I rank it under. In short, it must not be entirely new, but have something in it old and already perceived by me. It must, I say, have so much at least in common with the ideas I have before known and named as to

make me give it the same name with them. But it has been, if I mistake not, clearly made out that a man born blind would not at first reception of his sight think the things he saw were of the same nature with the objects of touch, or had anything in common with them; but that they were a new set of ideas, perceived in a new manner, and entirely different from all he had ever perceived before: so that he would not call them by the same name, nor repute them to be of the same sort with anything he had hitherto known.

129. SECONDLY, light and colours are allowed by all to constitute a son or species entirely different from the ideas of touch: nor will any man, I presume, say they can make themselves perceived by that sense: but there is no other immediate object of sight besides light and colours. It is therefore a direct consequence that there is no idea common to both senses.

130. It is a prevailing opinion, even amongst those who have thought and writ most accurately concerning our ideas and the ways whereby they enter into the understanding, that something more is perceived by sight than barely light and colours with their variations. Mr. Locke termeth sight, 'The most comprehensive of all our senses, conveying to our minds the ideas of light and colours, which are peculiar only to that sense; and also the far different ideas of space, figure, and motion. ESSAY ON HUMAN UNDERSTAND. B. ii. C. 9. S. 9. Space or distance, we have shown, is not otherwise the object of sight than of hearing. VID. sect. 46. And as for figure and extension, I leave it to anyone that shall calmly attend to his own clear and distinct ideas to decide whether he had any idea intromitted immediately and properly by sight save only light and colours: or whether it De possible for him to frame in his mind a distinct abstract idea of visible extension or figure exclusive of all colour: and on the other hand, whether he can conceive colour without visible extension? For my own part, I must confess I am not able to attain so great a nicety of abstraction: in a strict sense, I see nothing but light and colours, with their several shades and variations. He who beside these doth also perceive by sight ideas far different and distinct from them hath that faculty in a degree more perfect and comprehensive than I can pretend to. It must be owned that by the mediation of light and colours other far different ideas are suggested to my mind: but so they are by hearing, which beside sounds which are peculiar to that sense, doth by their mediation suggest not only space, figure, and motion, but also all other ideas whatsoever that can be signified by words.

131. THIRDLY, it is, I think, an axiom universally received that quantities of the same kind may be added together and make one entire sum. Mathematicians add lines together: but they do not add a line to a solid, or conceive it as making one sum with a surface: these three kinds of quantity being thought incapable of any such mutual addition, and consequently of being compared together in the several ways of proportion, are by then esteemed entirely disparate and heterogeneous. Now let anyone try in his thoughts to add a visible line or surface to a tangible line or surface, so as to conceive them making one continued sum or whole. He that can do this may think them homogeneous: but he that cannot, must by the foregoing axiom think them heterogeneous. A blue and a red line I can conceive added together into one sum and making one continued line: but to make in my thoughts one continued line of a visible and tangible line added together is, I find, a task far more difficult, and even insurmountable: and I leave it to the reflexion and experience of every particular person to determine for himself.

132. A farther confirmation of our tenet may be drawn from the solution of Mr. Molyneux's problem, published by Mr. Locke in his ESSAY: which I shall set down as it there lies, together with Mr. Locke's opinion of it, '"Suppose a man born blind, and now adult, and taught by his touch to distinguish between a cube and a sphere of the same metal, and nighly [SIC] of the same bigness, so as to tell, when he felt one and t'other, which is the cube and which the sphere. Suppose then the cube and sphere placed on a table, and the blind man to be made to see: QUAERE, whether by his sight, before he touched them, he could now distinguish and tell which is the globe, which the cube?" To which the acute and judicious proposer answers: "Not. For though he has obtained the experience of how a globe, how a cube, affects his touch, yet he has not yet attained the experience that what affects his touch so or so must affect his sight so or so: or that a protuberant angle in the cube that pressed his hand unequally shall appear to his eye as it doth in the cube." I agree with this thinking gentleman, whom I am proud to call my friend, in his answer to this his problem; and am of opinion that the blind man at first sight would not be able with certainty to say which was the globe, which the cube, whilst he only saw them.' (ESSAY ON HUMAN UNDERSTANDING, B. ii. C. 9. S. 8.)

133. Now, if a square surface perceived by touch be of the same sort with a square surface perceived by sight, it is certain the blind man here mentioned might know a square surface as soon as he saw it: it is no more but introducing into his mind by a new inlet an idea he has been already well acquainted with. Since, therefore, he is supposed to have known by his touch that a cube is a body terminated by square surfaces, and that a

sphere is not terminated by square surfaces: upon the supposition that a visible and tangible square differ only IN NUMERO it follows that he might know, by the unerring mark of the square surfaces, which was the cube, and which not, while he only saw them. We must therefore allow either that visible extension and figures are specifically distinct from tangible extension and figures, or else that the solution of this problem given by those two thoughtful and ingenious men is wrong.

134. Much more might be laid together in proof of the proposition I have advanced: but what has been said is, if I mistake not, sufficient to convince anyone that shall yield a reasonable attention: and as for those that will not be at the pains of a little thought, no multiplication of words will ever suffice to make them understand the truth, or rightly conceive my meaning.

135. I cannot let go the above–mentioned problem without some reflexion on it. It hath been evident that a man blind from his birth would not, at first sight, denominate anything he saw by the names he had been used to appropriate to ideas of touch, VID. sect. 106. Cube, sphere, table are words he has known applied to things perceivable by touch, but to things perfectly intangible he never knew them applied. Those words in their wonted application always marked out to his mind bodies or solid things which were perceived by the resistance they gave: but there is no solidity, no resistance or protrusion, perceived by sight. In short, the ideas of sight are all new perceptions, to which there be no names annexed in his mind: he cannot therefore understand what is said to him concerning them: and to ask of the two bodies he saw placed on the table, which was the sphere, which the cube? were to him a question downright bantering and unintelligible; nothing he sees being able to suggest to his thoughts the idea of body, distance, or in general of anything he had already known.

136. It is a mistake to think the same thing affects both sight and touch. If the same angle or square which is the object of touch be also the object of vision, what should hinder the blind man at first sight from knowing it? For though the manner wherein it affects the sight be different from that wherein it affected his touch, yet, there being beside his manner or circumstance, which is new and unknown, the angle or figure, which is old and known, he cannot choose but discern it.

137. Visible figure and extension having been demonstrated to be of a nature entirely different and heterogeneous from tangible figure and extension, it remains that we inquire

concerning. Now that visible motion is not of the same sort with tangible motion seems to need no farther proof, it being an evident corollary from what we have shown concerning the difference there is between visible and tangible extension: but for a more full and express proof hereof we need only observe that one who had not yet experienced vision would not at first sight know motion. Whence it clearly follows that motion perceivable by sight is of a sort distinct from motion perceivable by touch. The antecedent I prove thus: by touch he could not perceive any motion but what was up or down, to the right or left, nearer or farther from him; besides these and their several varieties or complications, it is impossible he should have any idea of motion. He would not therefore think anything to be motion, or give the name motion to any idea which he could not range under some or other of those particular kinds thereof. But from sect. 95 it is plain that by the mere act of vision he could not know motion upwards or downwards, to the right or left, or in any other possible direction. From which I conclude he would not know motion at all at first sight. As for the idea of motion in abstract, I shall not waste paper about it, but leave it to my reader to make the best he can of it. To me it is perfectly unintelligible.

138. The consideration of motion may furnish a new field for inquiry: but since the manner wherein the mind apprehends by sight the motion of tangible objects, with the various degrees thereof, may be easily collected from what hath been said concerning the manner wherein that sense doth suggest their various distances, magnitudes, and situations, I shall not enlarge any farther on this subject, but proceed to consider what may be alleged, with greatest appearance of reason, against the proposition we have shown to be true. For where there is so much prejudice to be encountered, a bare and naked demonstration of the truth will scarce suffice. We must also satisfy the scruples that men may raise in favour of their preconceived notions, show whence the mistake arises, how it came to spread, and carefully disclose and root out those false persuasions that an early prejudice might have implanted in the mind.

139. FIRST, therefore, it will be demanded how visible extension and figures come to be called by the same name with tangible extension and figures, if they are not of the same kind with them? It must be something more than humour or accident that could occasion a custom so constant and universal as this, which has obtained in all ages and nations of the world, and amongst allranks of men, the learned as well as the illiterate.

140. To which I answer, we can no more argue a visible and tangible square to be of the same species from their being called by the same name, than we can that a tangible

square and the monosyllable consisting of six letters whereby it is marked are of the same species because they are both called by the same name. It is customary to call written words and the things they signify by the same name: for words not being regarded in their own nature, or otherwise than as they are marks of things, it had been superfluous, and beside the design of language, to have given them names distinct from those of the things marked by them. The same reason holds here also. Visible figures are the marks of tangible figures, and from sect. 59 it is plain that in themselves they are little regarded, or upon any other score than for their connexion with tangible figures, which by nature they are ordained to signify. And because this language of nature doth not vary in different ages or nations, hence it is that in all times and places visible figures are called by the same names as the respective tangible figures suggested by them, and not because they are alike or of the same sort with them.

141. But, say you, surely a tangible square is liker to a visible square than to a visible circle: it has four angles and as many sides: so also has the visible square: but the visible circle has no such thing, being bounded by one uniform curve without right lines or angles, which makes it unfit to represent the tangible square but very fit to represent the tangible circle. Whence it clearly follows that visible figures are patterns of, or of the same species with, the respective tangible figures represented by them: that they are like unto them, and of their own nature fitted to represent them, as being of the same sort: and that they are in no respect arbitrary signs, as words.

142. I answer, it must be acknowledged the visible square is fitter than the visible circle to represent the tangible square, but then it is not because it is liker, or more of a species with it, but because the visible square contains in it several distinct parts, whereby to mark the several distinct corresponding parts of a tangible square, whereas the visible circle doth not. The square perceived by touch hath four distinct, equal sides, so also hath it four distinct equal angles. It is therefore necessary that the visible figure which shall be most proper to mark it contain four distinct equal parts corresponding to the four sides of the tangible square, as likewise four other distinct and equal parts whereby to denote the four equal angles of the tangible square. And accordingly we see the visible figures contain in them distinct visible parts, answering to the distinct tangible parts of the figures signified or suggested by them.

143. But it will not hence follow that any visible figure is like unto, or of the same species with, its corresponding tangible figure, unless it be also shown that not only the

number but also the kind of the parts be the same in both. To illustrate this, I observe that visible figures represent tangible figures much after the same manner that written words do sounds. Now, in this respect words are not arbitrary, it not being indifferent what written word stands for any sound: but it is requisite that each word contain in it so many distinct characters as there are variations in the sound it stands for. Thus the single letter A is proper to mark one simple uniform sound; and the word ADULTERY is accommodated to represent the sound annexed to it, in the formation whereof there being eight different collisions or modifications of the air by the organs of speech, each of which produces a difference of sound, it was fit the word representing it should consist of as many distinct characters, thereby to mark each particular difference or part of the whole sound. And yet nobody, I presume, will say the single letter a, or the word ADULTERY, are like unto, or of the same species with, the respective sounds by them represented. It is indeed arbitrary that, in general, letters of any language represent sounds at all: but when that is once agreed, it is not arbitrary what combination of letters shall represent this or that particular sound. I leave this with the reader to pursue, and apply it in his own thoughts.

144. It must be confessed that we are not so apt to confound other signs with the things signified, or to think them of the same species, as we are visible and tangible ideas. But a little consideration will show us how this may be without our supposing them of a like nature. These signs are constant and universal, their connexion with tangible ideas has been learnt at our first entrance into the world; and ever since, almost every moment of our lives, it has been occurring to our thoughts, and fastening and striking deeper on our minds. When we observe that signs are variable, and of human institution; when we remember there was a time they were not connected in our minds with those things they now so readily suggest; but that their signification was learned by the slow steps of experience: this preserves us from confounding them. But when we find the same signs suggest the same things all over the world; when we know they are not of human institution, and cannot remember that we ever learned their signification, but think that at first sight they would have suggested to us the same things they do now: all this persuades us they are of the same species as the things respectively represented by them, and that it is by a natural resemblance they suggest them to our minds.

145. Add to this that whenever we make a nice survey of any object, successively directing the optic axis to each point thereof, there are certain lines and figures described by the motion of the head or eye, which being in truth perceived by feeling, do

nevertheless so mix themselves, as it were, with the ideas of sight, that we can scarce think but they appertain to that sense. Again, the ideas of sight enter into the mind several at once, more distinct and unmingled than is usual in the other senses beside the touch. Sounds, for example, perceived at the same instant, are apt to coalesce, if I may so say, into one sound: but we can perceive at the same time great variety of visible objects, very separate and distinct from each other. Now tangible extension being made up of several distinct coexistent parts, we may hence gather another reason that may dispose us to imagine a likeness or an analogy between the immediate objects of sight and touch. But nothing, certainly, doth more contribute to blend and confound them together than the strict and close connexion they have with each other. We cannot open our eyes but the ideas of distance, bodies, and tangible figures are suggested by them. So swift and sudden and unperceived is the transition from visible to tangible ideas that we can scarce forbear thinking them equally the immediate object of vision.

146. The prejudice which is grounded on these, and whatever other causes may be assigned thereof, sticks so fast that it is impossible without obstinate striving and labour of the mind to get entirely clear of it. But then the reluctancy we find in rejecting any opinion can be no argument of its truth to whoever considers what has been already shown with regard to the prejudices we entertain concerning the distance, magnitude, and situation of objects; prejudices so familiar to our minds, so confirmed and inveterate, as they will hardly give way to the clearest demonstration.

147. Upon the whole, I think we may fairly conclude that the proper objects of vision constitute an universal language of the Author of Nature, whereby we are instructed how to regulate our actions in order to attain those things that are necessary to the preservation and well–being of our bodies, as also to avoid whatever may be hurtful and destructive of them. It is by their information that we are principally guided in all the transactions and concerns of life. And the manner wherein they signify and mark unto us the objects which are at a distance is the same with that of languages and signs of human appointment, which do not suggest the things signified by any likeness or identity of nature, but only by an habitual connexion that experience has made us to observe between them.

148. Suppose one who had always continued blind be told by his guide that after he has advanced so many steps he shall come to the brink of a precipice, or be stopped by a wall; must not this to him seem very admirable and surprizing? He cannot conceive how

it is possible for mortals to frame such predictions as these, which to him would seem as strange and unaccountable as prophesy doth to others. Even they who are blessed with the visive faculty may (though familiarity make it less observed) find therein sufficient cause of admiration. The wonderful art and contrivance wherewith it is adjusted to those ends and purposes for which it was apparently designed, the vast extent, number, and variety of objects that are at once with so much ease and quickness and pleasure suggested by it: all these afford subject for much and pleasing speculation, and may, if anything, give us some glimmering analogous prenotion of things which are placed beyond the certain discovery and comprehension of our present state.

149. I do not design to trouble myself with drawing corollaries from the doctrine I have hitherto laid down. If it bears the test others may, so far as they shall think convenient, employ their thoughts in extending it farther, and applying it to whatever purposes it may be subservient to: only, I cannot forbear making some inquiry concerning the object of geometry, which the subject we have been upon doth naturally lead one to. We have shown there is no such idea as that of extension in abstract, and that there are two kinds of sensible extension and figures which are entirely distinct and heterogeneous from each other. Now, it is natural to inquire which of these is the object of geometry.

150. Some things there are which at first sight incline one to think geometry conversant about visible extension. The constant use of the eyes, both in the practical and speculative parts of that science, doth very much induce us thereto. It would, without doubt, seem odd to a mathematician to go about to convince him the diagrams he saw upon paper were not the figures, or even the likeness of the figures, which make the subject of the demonstration. The contrary being held an unquestionable truth, not only by mathematicians, but also by those who apply themselves more particularly to the study of logic; I mean, who consider the nature of science, certainty, and demonstration: it being by them assigned as one reason of the extraordinary clearness and evidence of geometry that in this science the reasonings are free from those inconveniences which attend the use of arbitrary signs, the very ideas themselves being copied out and exposed to view upon paper. But, by the bye, how well this agrees with what they likewise assert of abstract ideas being the object of geometrical demonstration I leave to be considered.

151. To come to a resolution in this point we need only observe what hath been said in sect. 59, 60, 61, where it is shown that visible extensions in themselves are little regarded, and have no settled determinable greatness, and that men measure altogether, by the

application of tangible extension to tangible extension. All which makes it evident that visible extension and figures are not the object of geometry.

152. It is therefore plain that visible figure are of the same use in geometry that words are: and the one may as well be accounted the object of that science as the other, neither of them being otherwise concerned therein than as they represent or suggest to the mind the particular tangible figures connected with them. There is indeed this difference between the signification of tangible figures by visible figures, and of ideas by words: that whereas the latter is variable and uncertain, depending altogether on the arbitrary appointment of men, the former is fixed and immutably the same in all times and places. A visible square, for instance, suggests to the mind the same tangible figure in Europe that it doth in America. Hence it is that the voice of the Author of Nature which speaks to our eyes, is not liable to that misinterpretation and ambiguity that languages of human contrivance are unavoidably subject to.

153. Though what has been said may suffice to show what ought to be determined with relation to the object of geometry, I shall nevertheless, for the fuller illustration thereof, consider the case of an intelligence, or unbodied spirit, which is supposed to see perfectly well, i.e. to have a clear perception of the proper and immediate objects of sight, but to have no sense of touch. Whether there be any such being in Nature or no is beside my purpose to inquire. It sufficeth that the supposition contains no contradiction in it. Let us now examine what proficiency such a one may be able to make in geometry. Which speculation will lead us more clearly to see whether the ideas of sight can possibly be the object of that science.

154. FIRST, then, it is certain the aforesaid intelligence could have no idea of a solid, or quantity of three dimensions, which followeth from its not having any idea of distance. We indeed are prone to think that we have by sight the ideas of space and solids, which ariseth from our imagining that we do, strictly speaking, see distance and some parts of an object at a greater distance than others; which hath been demonstrated to be the effect of the experience we have had, what ideas of touch are connected with such and such ideas attending vision: but the intelligence here spoken of is supposed to have no experience of touch. He would not, therefore, judge as we do, nor have any idea of distance, outness, or profundity, nor consequently of space or body, either immediately or by suggestion. Whence it is plain he can have no notion of those parts of geometry which relate to the mensuration of solids and their convex or concave surfaces, and contemplate

the properties of lines generated by the section of a solid. The conceiving of any part whereof is beyond the reach of his faculties.

155. Farther, he cannot comprehend the manner wherein geometers describe a right line or circle; the rule and compass with their use being things of which it is impossible he should have any notion: nor is it an easier matter for him to conceive the placing of one plane or angle on another, in order to prove their equality: since that supposeth some idea of distance or external space. All which makes it evident our pure intelligence could never attain to know so much as the first elements of plane geometry. And perhaps upon a nice inquiry it will be found he cannot even have an idea of plane figures any more than he can of solids; since some idea of distance is necessary to form the idea of a geometrical plane, as will appear to whoever shall reflect a little on it.

156. All that is properly perceived by the visive faculty amounts to no more than colours, with their variations and different proportions of light and shade. But the perpetual mutability and fleetingness of those immediate objects of sight render them incapable of being managed after the manner of geometrical figures; nor is it in any degree useful that they should. It is true there are divers of them perceived at once, and more of some and less of others: but accurately to compute their magnitude and assign precise determinate proportions between things so variable and inconstant, if we suppose it possible to be done, must yet be a very trifling and insignificant labour.

157. I must confess men are tempted to think that flat or plane figures are immediate objects of sight, though they acknowledge solids are not. And this opinion is grounded on what is observed in painting, wherein (it seems) the ideas immediately imprinted on the mind are only of planes variously coloured, which by a sudden act of the judgment are changed into solids. But with a little attention we shall find the planes here mentioned as the immediate objects of sight are not visible but tangible planes. For when we say that pictures are planes, we mean thereby that they appear to the touch smooth and uniform. But then this smoothness and uniformity, or, in other words, this planeness of the picture, is not perceived immediately by vision: for it appeareth to the eye various and multiform.

158. From all which we may conclude that planes are no more the immediate object of sight than solids. What we strictly see are not solids, nor yet planes variously coloured: they are only diversity of colours. And some of these suggest to the mind solids, and other plane figures, just as they have been experienced to be connected with the one or

the other: so that we see planes in the same way that we see solids, both being equally suggested by the immediate objects of sight, which accordingly are themselves denominated planes and solids. But though they are called by the same names with the things marked by them, they are nevertheless of a nature entirely different, as hath been demonstrated.

159. What hath been said is, if I mistake not, sufficient to decide the question we proposed to examine, concerning the ability of a pure spirit, such as we have described, to know GEOMETRY. It is, indeed, no easy matter for us to enter precisely into the thoughts of such an intelligence, because we cannot without great pains cleverly separate and disentangle in our thoughts the proper objects of sight from those of touch which are connected with them. This, indeed, in a complete degree seems scarce possible to be performed: which will not seem strange to us if we consider how hard it is for anyone to hear the words of his native language pronounced in his ears without understanding them. Though he endeavour to disunite the meaning from the sound, it will nevertheless intrude into his thoughts, and he shall find it extreme difficult, if not impossible, to put himself exactly in the posture of a foreigner that never learned the language, so as to be affected barely with the sounds themselves, and not perceive the signification annexed to them.

160. By this time, I suppose, it is clear that neither abstract nor visible extension makes the object of geometry; the not discerning of which may perhaps have created some difficulty and useless labour in mathematics. Sure I am, that somewhat relating thereto has occurred to my thoughts, which, though after the most anxious and repeated examination I am forced to think it true, doth, nevertheless, seem so far out of the common road of geometry, that I know not whether it may not be thought presumption, if I should make it public in an age, wherein that science hath received such mighty improvements by new methods; great part whereof, as well as of the ancient discoveries, may perhaps lose their reputation, and much of that ardour with which men study the abstruse and fine geometry be abated, if what to me, and those few to whom I have imparted it, seems evidently true, should really prove to be so.

Printed in the United States
23805LVS00002B/63-84